Eating with Purpose

Keep it Healthy, Keep it Simple, Keep it Delicious

Vicki Twiford

ACKNOWLEDGMENTS

This book is dedicated to my family:

♦ To my husband Don who began eating healthy just to support me. His patience, during both my research and the writing of this book, was a tremendous encouragement to me.
♦ To my children, Danae and Donny: I pray this notebook will inspire them to eat healthy to make up for all of the years that I didn't know about eating for health and healing.

I want to thank Rachelle Colgrove, Molly Benson and Pat Ashby for the hours they spent editing; Sharon Buck, Lois Hostettler, and Judy Gauntt for their testimonies which inspired me to do research which led to my own healing; and Teri North for advising me as a health coach.

The majority of information in this notebook is what I learned from the following resources:

The Maker's Diet by Jordan S. Rubin N.M.D., Ph.D.; Joseph Brasco, M.D.

(Recommended by **Dr. Charles F. Stanley**, Senior Pastor, First Baptist Church, Atlanta, Georgia, Founder and President, In Touch Ministries)

Toxic Relief by Don Colbert, M.D.

(Recommended by **Rev. John Hagee**, Pastor, Cornerstone Church, San Antonio, Texas)

What the Bible Says About Healthy Living by Rex Russell, M.D.

(Recommended by **Dr. Bill Bright**, Founder and President, Campus Crusade for Christ International; **Larry Burkett**, President and Founder, Christian Financial Concepts)

Prescription for Nutritional Healing by Phyllis A. Balch, C.N.C.; James F. Balch, M.D.

(Most health food stores rely on this book as a reference tool when recommending supplements.)

For a complete list of resources, see the *Resource List* on the last page of this notebook.

ENDORSEMENTS

What a joy to hear Vicki share her testimony and life decisions concerning health and eating wisely. Her approach was simple, faith-building, and easy for others to understand and engage as new habits in their life. Her love for Christ, for others, and for the body of Christ to live well is very evident. She is a good communicator and handles her audience with clarity and purpose. Your groups will enjoy this time of teaching and be encouraged to live healthy so the gospel and glory of Christ will be revealed in their lives.

(Rev. Joy Headley, Family Pastor, Gospel Lighthouse Church, Dallas, Texas)

I began a journey of weight loss several years ago without an understanding of food and its importance for a healthy body. After attending the Health Seminar with Vicki, food became my friend instead of my enemy. This has changed EVERYTHING for me. I now embrace God's plan for me and my family to be healthy and happy. Vicki presents her case for living life to its fullest through diet in a very practical, upbeat, easy to understand manner. The women of our church were inspired by sitting under Vicki's teaching, and are on the path to leading their families into wholeness: body, soul and spirit.

(Becky Hennesy, Director of Women's Ministry, Trinity Church, Cedar Hill, Texas)

What this notebook is:

This notebook is a compilation of the notes that I took while reading the materials listed on the resource page. As I read these books, I discovered that not all nutritionists and doctors agree on every issue concerning what we should and should not eat. So I spent several months trying to sort out what might be a general consensus. At the same time, I discovered that God put specific nutrients in food that were meant for our health and our healing. Therefore, I restricted inclusion in this notebook to the following:

1.   Information that I felt did not contradict scripture.

2.   Information about which there was a general consensus among the authors I read.

3.   Instructions I could reasonably follow without having to find some unusual food item.

My personal motto is: Keep it Healthy, Keep it Simple, Keep it Delicious

I gave these notes to my family so they would not have to spend the same amount of time doing their own research. We all wanted to change our eating habits and be in better health. As other people noticed a difference in our health, they began asking me for a copy of my notes. I put the notes into my own words and formatted them into easy to read charts. What you are about to read is the result. **Note: Blank pages are included for recording research on each topic concerning your own health issues.**

What this notebook is not:

Disclaimer: I am not a nutritionist or a doctor. These notes are not intended to be used as medical advice and you should always consult your health care provider concerning health decisions. The information concerning the healing powers of food is simply from my research. My personal advice concerning eating healthy is always indicated as such and is written in this notebook for informational purposes only, as well as advice directed to my family only. Please realize, my personal notations are from the perspective of a homemaker as an incentive for my own family to eat healthier (and should be taken as such).

By reading this notebook, you acknowledge that you are responsible for your own health decisions. Any statements or claims about the possible health benefits conferred by any foods or supplements have not been evaluated by the Food & Drug Administration and are not intended to diagnose, treat, cure or prevent any disease.

This notebook is also not intended as a diet recommendation to lose weight, although I have lost and maintained a healthy weight by eating in this manner. For a healthy diet for losing weight, I would recommend Beyonddiet.com.

No portion of this notebook may be re-printed without express written permission of the author. (Exception: License is given to make a single copy of pages where it is recommended for personal use.)

Table of Contents

1 - My Personal Journey

In our travels as evangelists, my husband and I came in contact with pastors and their wives from four different states who had experienced a physical healing in their bodies through changing their diet and doing a cleanse (see chapter 5). I was skeptical at first. Then, we spoke with one pastor's wife who at one time had been in excruciating pain from arthritis. She was unable to sleep at night or pick up her own grandchildren without great pain. However, she experienced healing through a diet change, juicing, and supplements. I decided to purchase some books by respected doctors and nutritionists and do my own research.

The results were far beyond what I had expected. Little did I know that scientific research about the chemicals contained in food would enhance my understanding about the love of God. For instance (as you will learn in Chapter 4) there are chemicals God created in fruits and vegetables that defend, fight for, and cleanse the living cells in our body. This brought new light to Roman 1:20 which tells us that God's physical creation helps us to understand His invisible qualities. He is certainly my defender and the one who sustains my life!

Another illustration is found in the Passover meal. When the Israelites came out of Egypt, they were instructed by God to eat bitter herbs. While not all bitter herbs were created for food, there are numerous herbs which both cleanse and heal the body. According to Dr. Russell, herbs were used for this purpose not only by the Hebrews, but also by the Egyptians, Persians, and Chinese (1996. 201). These herbs were so powerful that ancient people thought there were spirits inside the herbs that healed their bodies. What they didn't understand was that God created these foods as proof of His desire for our health.

The evidence was so convincing that I decided to change my own eating habits. My husband did the same just to support me. At the time, I had miserable allergies, headaches, and joint pains. After just four months, the allergies were gone, I no longer had constant headaches, and the joint pain disappeared. As a bonus, I felt like my brain "woke up." To top it all off, my husband lost 35 pounds and I lost 14 pounds without even trying.

Does that mean we no longer rely upon God for a supernatural healing? On the contrary, both my husband and I have experienced miraculous healing through the power of prayer. But now, our faith has been enriched by the six months of research contained in this notebook. I have come to see a fuller revelation of God as my healer. Deuteronomy 6:1-2 says that God wants us to "**enjoy long life**". Proverbs 4:20-22 says, he wants to bring, "**health to a man's whole body**" Proverbs 3:7-8 says his ways "**bring health to your body and nourishment to your bones.**" Yet, I had never considered this as having anything to do with what we eat. That is, until I did my homework and changed my eating habits.

Jordan Rubin, author of "Restoring Your Digestive Health" says that although America is a technologically advanced nation, out of thirteen nations studied, we rank next to the last on health issues. Imagine what a testimony it would be to the rest of the world if God's people lived in health today. They would be asking us what we're doing differently. That doesn't mean we will never be ill. We live in a sin cursed world. But we can certainly be on the offensive through prayer and attentiveness to God's Word.

I pray that after reading this notebook, when you sit down to a plate full of bright colored vegetables, you'll truly thank God for what He has given you for health. I pray that you will no longer look at food simply as a means to get full; but instead, you will look at food as the abundant supply of our loving heavenly Father for the health of your body. Enjoy!

Notes (write down health issues you would like to change)

4

2 - How Poor Eating Habits Can Lead to Disease

Most of us are familiar with the fact that bacteria and viruses can get into our bodies and cause us to become ill. We are also familiar with the fact that air pollutants and carcinogens can attack cells in our bodies, leading to diseases such as cancer. Understanding how that happens can give us more of an incentive to eat healthy.

Every molecule in the cells of our body contains electrons. Every cell will seek to have a balanced number of electrons. When something damages a cell, causing it to lose an electron, the damaged cell will act like a wrecking ball, trying to rob other cells of electrons to balance itself. These unbalanced cells are called Free Radicals and can start a chain reaction. Some of these cells may oxidize (like an apple turning brown). Depending on which cells are damaged, they may lead to common complaints such as a lack of energy, fatigue, foggy brain, depression, a depressed metabolism, food cravings, cellulite, constipation, and acne. They may also lead to more serious diseases such as cancer, ALS, Alzheimer's, Atherosclerosis, Diabetes, and Parkinson's.

God designed our bodies to handle a certain amount of free radicals which occur naturally. He also designed the body to ward off a certain number of pollutants. However, excesses can be caused by cigarette smoke, processed foods, food additives, fried foods, pollutants, radiation, infections, and abuse of drugs. The good news is that pollutants and free radicals can be fought by the nutrients which God put in food. That is, if we eat right. The goal is to have more God-given nutrients going into your body than you have free radicals. Dr. Rex Russell, in *What the Bible Says About Healthy Living*, suggests that if we follow three basic principles (as much as possible) we will be well on our way to better health. Two of his principles are mentioned in this chapter:

1.   **Eat foods as they were created** (without chemical additives or laboratory refinement)

2.   **Don't make any food your god** (1996. 29)

Dr. Russell's 3rd principal applies to "clean and unclean animals," and advises eating only what God gave us for food. I personally struggled with this issue. The truth is, Jesus said, "Don't you see that nothing that enters a man from the outside can make him 'unclean'? For it doesn't go into his heart but into his stomach, and then out of his body." (In saying this, Jesus declared all foods "clean." Mark 7:18-19) In addition, animals are raised in much cleaner conditions today. (For further research on this issue, as well as my personal view, see Appendix A.)

Regardless of where you stand on this issue, as evidenced by the health concerns in America today, there is definitely room for improvement. With the invention of the supermarket introducing processed foods, and the demand of our busy schedules, the health of America began to deteriorate. It is only recently that we have begun to realize that this modernization has contributed to many illnesses. The notes in this chapter show how this is true. But don't get too discouraged, chapters three and four offer great hope.

The solution is really quite easy. In fact, I have found that cooking healthy is much easier than I had thought. It just takes a little time to adjust old habits. It also takes time to adjust our thinking, or at least it did mine. To begin, as you read this chapter, use the "Notes" page at the end of this chapter and/or the "My Plan" sheet in Appendix C to list foods you may need to omit from your diet. It is also advisable that, when devising a plan, you should take into consideration your own health issues, the medical history of your family, and consult with your doctor. Some people will need to make more changes than others. Also, blank pages are included for the purpose of taking notes as you read and develop your own plan.

Principle 1. Eating foods that man has altered may lead to disease.

Hydrogenated fats are currently being looked at as a leading cause of many diseases. When man changes liquid oil into a solid by the process of hydrogenation, it causes a chemical change in the oil that results in what is called trans-fats. Two examples are shortening and margarine. These trans-fats become part of our cell membranes. When an altered trans-fat gets into the cell membrane, it weakens the outer lining of the cell. This leaves the cell vulnerable to attack and deterioration. Trans-fats are also caused by heating unstable vegetable oils. They can raise bad cholesterol, acting the same as bacon grease in a drain. Trans-fats may lead to arthritis, cancer, Crohn's disease, high blood pressure, coronary heart disease, and acne. They're being looked at as the biggest health disaster of our time. Warning labels are beginning to appear on many foods. Unfortunately, many processed foods have hydrogenated oils in them. French fries, margarine, shortening, most potato chips, doughnuts, and cake all contain trans-fats. Butter and olive oil have no trans-fats.

Hormones and antibiotics given to animals through injection go into the meat that ends up in our stomachs. Some doctors believe this is the reason so many people are allergic to antibiotics, and many women have a hormone imbalance (uncommon in other countries). These same substances are found in the milk and cheese from cows that are not organically raised.

Nitrates used in cold cuts, bacon, ham, and even smoked fish may create free radicals.

Herbicides and pesticides on fruits and vegetables attack our cells and may create free radicals.

Aspartame may act as a neurotoxin and cause brain tumors, headaches, fatigue, dizziness, nausea, blurred vision, and depression. Aspartame is in many diet products, chewing gums, and breath mints.

Sucralose may weaken the immune system and cause bladder or kidney problems.

Pasteurization causes altered proteins. It also destroys the vitamins in the milk. Non-organic milk can also contain numerous antibiotics which may lead to antibiotic-resistant bacteria in your body. It also has more calcium than magnesium. Because the body needs magnesium to absorb calcium, the body will take magnesium from the body to absorb the calcium, leaving magnesium depletion. This may lead to calcium deposits, heart conditions, backaches, muscle tightness, and general tension.

Refined sugar turns immediately to glucose in your body which, in abundance, turns to fat. One coke can contain ten teaspoons of sugar. Although you need "good" sugars for energy, refined white sugar depletes the body of nutrients and feeds some bacteria. Too much refined sugar can result in hypoglycemia, obesity, behavioral disorders, yeast problems, and a decreased immune system. Eating just a few doughnuts reduces the body's ability to destroy micro-organisms for several hours. This could leave you susceptible to bacteria and viruses during that time.

Refined white flour is another major cause of obesity. It turns to glucose quickly in your system. It is bleached and processed, depleting it of vitamins. The outer husk of the wheat is where the vitamins are and it is removed in the making of white flour.

Overcooked vegetables are depleted of many vitamins. Heating food higher than 107 degrees may kill the natural enzymes put in them by God to help us with digestion.

Principle 1 Continued:

Harmful substances man adds to water, or are in our environment, include the following:

Chlorine can destroy certain vitamins. It may also form a chemical that causes cancer, allergies, asthma, and kidney stones.

Fluoride can inhibit enzymes in the body. Enzymes help our bodies with metabolism and digestion.

Aluminum is found in underarm deodorant, cookware, and aluminum foil. It may contribute to Alzheimer's, dementia, skin rashes, intestinal upset, and may be harmful to the bones and kidneys.

Mercury can be found in water and may cause numerous health problems.

Arsenic can come from ocean food, weed killer, and insecticides causing kidney problems, heart trouble, and damage to blood cells.

Lead can be found in water, some paints, food, and some cosmetics. Lead gets into the brain and nerves and may hamper memory, cause hyperactivity, learning disability, muscle pains, anemia, or poor digestion.

WHAT I CHOSE TO DO: Eat everything as our Creator gave it to us. In other words, I bought fresh instead of canned or packaged as much as possible.

Shop around the outside of the grocery store first. If I needed something like mayo, a processed food from an inside aisles, I looked for it in the health food section first or read the label to make sure it's natural.

I read all labels and bought only those products which have no hydrogenated or partially hydrogenated oils.

I bought free range meats as much as possible (meat from animals that have been raised in open fields, fed naturally, and given no hormones or antibiotics).

Getting raw milk can be difficult but some nutritionists highly recommend it. I did not make this switch. But some people found it necessary to switch to raw milk, goat's milk, or organic milk. We do however use coconut milk for things like oatmeal. I increased other foods high in calcium and magnesium (see chapter 4).

As much as possible, I bought organic vegetables and fruits. I rinsed them thoroughly (you can also use a vegetable wash).

To compensate for enzymes lost in the processing and cooking of vegetables I purchased enzyme supplements.

I went off chemical sweeteners. I used mostly honey or Stevia. The FDA has determined that aspartame is safe for human consumption, but this is disputed by many nutritionists

For bread, I ate whole grains and Ezekiel Bread which is available in most supermarkets. I drank filtered water. I have found reverse osmosis is best.

I changed from aluminum cookware and I avoided antiperspirants with aluminum.

Principle 2. Food addictions or fad diets that emphasize one food group can lead to disease.

Limiting certain foods which were given to us by God to nourish and protect our bodies may cause an imbalance of nutrients in our bodies. Many nutrients work synergistically and leaving one out can deplete our bodies of needed vitamins, minerals, amino acids, antioxidants, and enzymes. Going on a meat only diet may leave our bodies without the protection of antioxidants found in fruits and vegetables (see chapter 3). Meat in excess may lower the pH of tissues, cells can become acidic and can't release toxic waste from your body. On the other hand, eating no meat may leave the body without essential amino acids needed to build muscle and boost the immune system.

Caffeine in excess can cause a hormone imbalance. It may also lead to weight gain. It also reduces the absorption of iron into the body and may cause dehydration.

Salt in excess can cause high blood pressure. Processed foods often contain high amounts of salt.

WHAT I CHOSE TO DO: Follow the Creator's plan for eating a variety of foods and eat them in balance. (Covered more fully in the following chapters.) Use sea salt – it contains minerals like magnesium, calcium, potassium, sulfate, and several trace minerals.

In addition to violating the above two principles mentioned by Dr. Russell, the following abuses may also lead to disease.

Junk food may give us a full feeling due to bulk, but it may leave us depleted of nutrients and craving more food. God designed our body to get hungry when we need nutrients. When we eat, the brain sends a signal to the body to digest the food so it can receive the nutrients in the food. But when it finds no nutrients in the food, it keeps sending hunger signals, thus laboring your digestive tract without nutrients being supplied to the body. So the body keeps wanting more food because it is not finding nutrients in what you are eating. The phosphorus in soda pop actually depletes the body of calcium and your body will want more.

WHAT I CHOSE TO DO: Avoid junk food. Order a salad and eat sandwiches open faced with vegetables.

Overuse of manmade drugs and medications can overwhelm the liver. As you will see in the following chapters, God gave us food not only for nourishment, but for the healing of our bodies. God placed healing chemicals in herbs, vegetables, fruits, and oils. Herbs were once used to treat illnesses. However, with modernization we have invented chemical clones in laboratories. These synthetic clones are not easily processed by our body and can have harmful side effects because they were not made by God for consumption. Aspirin and antibiotics are common laboratory clones of natural substances.

WHAT I CHOSE TO DO: I chose to not take over-the-counter medicines unless I absolutely needed it. I also consulted with my doctor and health coach to see if I could switch to an alternative medicine such as herbs. I also found a nutritionist at a health food store who was willing to advise me concerning natural remedies.

Contamination in the air can lead to disease. Toxins from the air (as well as our food) take up residence in the fatty tissue of our bodies including the brain, lungs, and joints. Toxins include things we clean with in our homes. The result can be fatigue, headaches, allergies, mucus, bronchitis, acne, foggy thinking, food allergies, saggy skin, joint aches, arthritis, skin disorders, or a poor immune function.

WHAT I CHOSE TO DO: Make sure the air filter is clean in our home. I also do my best to get outside to breathe some fresh air.

Negative emotions can lead to disease. Hatred, jealousy, fear, anxiety, anger, and depression can cause adrenaline levels to rise which causes blood pressure to increase. It can interfere with digestion, suppress the immune system and decrease the body's ability to fight toxins. All of this can lead to high blood pressure, migraine headaches, heart disease, ulcers, fatigue, cancer, stroke, arthritis, or cancer.

WHAT I CHOSE TO DO: I did my best to not eat when I was upset. Forgiveness and laughter release in the brain chemicals called endorphins – similar to morphine – triggering a feeling of well-being throughout your entire body. Give your heart, liver, and lungs a treat – forgive and laugh.

Proverbs 17:22 *A cheerful heart is good medicine, but a crushed spirit dries up the bones.*
Proverbs 16:24 *Pleasant words are a honeycomb, sweet to the soul and healing to the bones.*

Poor digestion can lead to disease. No matter how many supplements you take, if you do not eat healthy your liver will be sluggish, affecting every organ in your body. Weight loss will be blocked as well. Blood flow may be restricted, hormones become unbalanced, vitamins are not processed, fat is not broken down, toxins are not processed and excreted and the immune system is overworked. All of this can lead to diseases such as cancer, arthritis, mental disorders, or diabetes. It can also result in obesity.

WHAT I CHOSE TO DO: Follow the guidelines in Chapter 5 for restoring digestive health.

Not letting the land rest in accordance with the Word of God can cause disease. Trace minerals come from the earth and are absorbed into plants which become our food. Our bodies do not produce them. Lack of crop rotation, not resting the soil, and over processing food means we do not get the minerals we need. The lack of trace minerals is compounded by the way we eat. For example, our bodies need a balance of phosphorus and calcium in the food we eat. Meat has a much higher level of phosphorus than calcium. It is helpful to eat something high in calcium, such broccoli, with your meat. Soda pop has phosphorus but no calcium, and may contribute to calcium depletion. This imbalance may also cause cravings. We turn to sugar and salt to satisfy those cravings.

WHAT I CHOSE TO DO: It would be helpful if more farmers went back to the Biblical principle of crop rotation. But since that it not the case, I just did my best to buy organic, eat a balanced meal, and not drink carbonated beverages.

Sin and attacks of Satan can cause disease. It must be said that, in addition to the physical causes of sickness, our bodies can suffer from the spiritual attacks of sin and Satan.

WHAT I CHOSE TO DO: No matter what the cause or the cure, our God is ALWAYS THE HEALER. Psalm 107:20 says, He sent His Word and healed them and rescued them from the grave. Prayer and the Word of God are always important to both our spiritual and physical well-being. Spend time with the Lord every morning in prayer and Bible reading.

Special Note: We are still in the process of making changes in our own lives. We took our family history into consideration, as well as our budget, and the availability of health foods. We realize it can be difficult. We travel frequently and are in small towns which have few choices for healthy food. So we do our best with what we have and pray. For more information on this subject I suggest you read "What You Don't Know May Be Killing You" by Doctor Colbert.

Notes (write down eating habits you plan to change)

80/20 Eating ↑ pollutants - hereditary, stress

Eat foods as they were created -

Don't make any food your God

Eliminate or decrease

Hydrogenated fats, additives (hormones - antibiotics, preservatives)

Artificial sweetners, refined foods, Caffeine, junk food

Glycemic load = how much of that food will

turn to glucose (simple sugar is high)

3 - Divine Health and Healing in…
Four Basic Food Nutrients

Since the creation of the world , God's invisible qualities- His eternal power and divine nature-
have been clearly seen,
being understood from what has been made, so that men are without excuse.
Romans 1:20

If you are anything like I was when I first started reading all this information, you might be feeling a little overwhelmed. However, this chapter presents great truths about the nutrients God put in food to protect us from disease and heal our bodies. For now, just think of setting two important goals for achieving better health. First, utilize the information in the previous chapter to **reduce the amount of toxins** going into your body. Then, use the information in the next two chapters to **increase the nutrients** going into your body which will protect it from unavoidable toxins. Every nutritionally sound food item that you put into your mouth is intended to bring health to your body. Last, unless you are chronically ill, you may want to **begin by making just a few changes each week.**

But for right now, simply read over this chapter and allow yourself to be awed by what God created for us in food. Everything that God made, including food, declares who He is. He made food, not just for us to enjoy and fill our stomachs, but to nourish our bodies, as well as help our bodies heal. God designed the body to heal itself. When you cut your finger, it heals with new skin. The same is true inside your body. If you feed your body the nutrients God gave you in accordance with His plan, your body will continually heal itself internally.

That does not mean food is a "cure all." In his book *The Maker's Diet*, Jordan Rubin says that genetics, environmental toxins, lifestyle choices, emotional and mental factors, and cultural trends all affect our health. But he also says that "diet remains the *single most influential factor in overall human health*" (2004. 32). The reason for this is that there are certain chemicals in food that are essential to man's well-being. Essential means that the body does not produce that nutrient on its own, so it is essential that we get it from an outside source.

This chapter includes charts with brief descriptions of the four basic food nutrients given to us by God to nourish and heal our bodies. These are often referred to as the macro-nutrients in food. In 1825, carbohydrates, protein, and fats were identified as the major components of food. Often neglected, however, is the fact that water is also a major nutrient needed by our body. In addition to these macro-nutrients, God also created micro-nutrients which will be discussed in Chapter 4.

A word of caution: When I first became aware of these magnificent truths, I kept trying to memorize everything and struggled with how to balance all of the nutrients. To say the least, it was a little overwhelming. I was defeating my purpose due to the stress I was causing myself. That is why I included Chapter 6 entitled Cooking Healthy Made Easy. For now, as you read Chapters 3 and 4, once again use the "Notes" page and "My Plan" sheet. List any foods and supplements you feel you may need to include in your diet.

Special Note: Some of the information in the following two chapters are my own brief lists compiled partly from reading books in the "Resource List", talking with nutritionists, and doing internet research.

THE FOUR BASIC FOOD NUTRIENTS (Macro-Nutrients)
GOD CREATED TO NOURISH OUR BODIES ARE:

1. Water
2. Carbohydrates
3. Protein (Amino Acids)
4. Fats/Oils (Fatty Acids)

1. WATER

Jesus answered her, "If you knew the gift of God and who it is that asks you for a drink, you would have asked him and he would have given you **living water** ." (John 4:10) A study of the physical benefits of water reveal some wonderful spiritual truths about our loving Heavenly Father.

What God created water to do for us	Eating with purpose
Transports nutrients in and out of cells. Increases the efficiency of the cells ability to carry nutrients. Transports waste out of cells and out of the body. Maintains body temperature.	Drink four large glasses a day (16 oz) or, eight small glasses (8 oz). A more concise measurement is to drink half of your body weight in ounces. Reverse osmosis is best. Do not drink within 30 minutes of meals – it dilutes digestive acids in the stomach so food is not broken down as well as it could be, and fewer nutrients are absorbed. Drink no more than 4 – 8 oz with a meal.

Informative Notes

The body has trillions of cells – many are replaced every year, literally remaking the body.

Most dead cells are flushed from the body through the kidneys – if you're drinking enough water

The organs in our body are made primarily of water. Not getting enough water may lead to the following medical conditions.

Muscles – asthma (not enough water in lung muscles)

Brain - Alzheimer's, foggy brain

Blood – high blood pressure

Bones – arthritis

Joint Cartilage – joint pain

Not enough water for the skin can lead to wrinkles. (Take water out of a plum and it turns to a prune – take water out of the skin and you get wrinkles.) Caffeine can cause you to lose water. (Colbert 2004. 27-33)

Dry mouth is just one of the signs of dehydration. Not enough water can lead to constipation. When you are constipated, toxins in your stools can be released back into your body. One of the first signs that the body is not being nourished is hard stools. You should have soft but formed stools at least two to three times a day (once for each meal). Drinking iced drinks with a meal may slow down digestive enzymes, so it is best to drink room temperature beverages.

Helpful Hints: We purchased a carbon water filter so we could drink tap water. The most highly recommended is reverse osmosis water which can be purchased at most grocery stores. Every morning we drink 16 ounces of room temperature water upon rising. After breakfast I fill another 16 ounce glass and drink it throughout the morning. After lunch and dinner I do the same.

2. CARBOHYDRATES

"I give you every seed-bearing plant on the face of the whole earth and every tree that has fruit with seed in it. They will be yours for food. (Genesis 2:8,9) Now the LORD God had planted a garden in the east, in Eden; and there he put the man he had formed. And the LORD God made all kinds of trees grow out of the ground — trees that were pleasing to the eye and good for food. (Genesis 1:29)

What God created carbohydrates to do for us	Eating with Purpose
All Carbohydrates turn into glucose in the body which is the major fuel for the body's cells, resulting in energy. However, there are some foods which convert quickly into glucose and jack up blood sugar. Then your blood sugar takes a nose dive and you get hungry and binge. High insulin levels also send a signal to your body which tells it to store fat. Insulin also prevents the breakdown of fat.	**Complex carbohydrates should be 40 percent of your calories (25 grams of fiber) which includes whole grains, vegetables, and fruits.**
Note: There's no such thing as a "bad" carbohydrate in its natural state. Only the carbohydrates which have been altered by man and are eaten in improper proportions are bad for you. Since we need the vitamins, minerals, and fiber from fruits, vegetables, and grains, it is important to limit refined sugar and white flour which are the true "bad" carbohydrates.	**Whole Grains** – Ezekiel Bread and stone ground whole wheat contain whole grains which bind the toxins in your digestive tract to remove them. They also provide needed bulk for stools. The healthiest (and least starchy) grains are: Ezekiel Bread, stone ground whole wheat, brown rice, oat bran, and millet.
	Vegetables and Fruits contain healthy carbohydrates, and are also full of nutrients and antioxidants. They also have fiber. The lowest carbohydrate fruits are berries, which also have the highest nutrient punch. Apples and oranges are also good. The highest carbohydrate fruits are bananas, prunes, and raisins.
Soluble Fiber absorbs toxins and fats lowering cholesterol throughout your body.	**Avoid, if not eliminate, refined white sugar and white flour.** Both of these turn quickly to glucose. Some diets suggest you go off grains for a period of time and rely on vegetables for fiber.
Insoluble Fiber passes through the digestive tract without being digested. It gives you a full feeling, cleanses the colon, and carries toxins out of the body. It also provides bulk for stools.	**Healthy fiber includes** broccoli, cauliflower, celery, lettuce, seeds, nuts, whole grains, beans, and ground flax. Vegetables have vitamins, antioxidants, and fiber.

Informative Notes: The term *glycemic index* is a measurement for how quickly a certain food turns into glucose in your body. The term *glycemic load* is a measurement for how much of that food turns to glucose. Bagels, sugar, and potatoes have both a high glycemic index and a high glycemic load. To find out the glycemic index and glycemic load of certain foods go to glycemicindex.com and click on GI Database.

Helpful Hints: I had a difficult time with fresh fruits and vegetables wilting before I would use them. I now buy many of them frozen (especially those used in cooking). I buy fresh for salads and snacking. Frozen is often healthier because it is picked ripe. Also, when storing fresh leafy greens, I wrap them in a paper towel and store them in a bag. I keep a bowl full of fresh fruit on the counter top, along with nuts for snacking. I use honey or raw sugar in place of refined sugar for many recipes. You can also use Stevia instead of sugar.

Note: I will sometimes use half whole wheat flour and half unbleached flour for a smoother texture in baking.

3. PROTEIN/Amino Acids (Includes meat – God is not a vegetarian)

(Genesis 9:2,3) *"Everything that lives and moves will be food for you. Just as I gave you the green plants, I now give you everything."* **According to Jordan Rubin, one reason why God added meat to the diet of the Israelites was because their labor had increased, therefore, they needed more protein for additional strength. In Acts 27:34, after a time of fasting, Paul said,** *"Wherefore I pray you to take some meat: for this is for your health."*

What God created protein to do for us	Eating with Purpose
When protein is broken down through digestion, the amino acids in the food become the building blocks for our bodies. Some amino acids are produced in our bodies. However, there are some which are not produced and must be consumed in food. **Complete Proteins** are foods which contain all of the essential amino acids (those not supplied in the body). **Incomplete Proteins** are foods which contain only some amino acids. Diets with little meat can combine foods to make a complete protein. Protein provides the body with energy, builds new cells, tissue, muscles, and raises metabolism. It also helps to manufacture hormones, antibodies, and enzymes. If you don't eat enough protein, the body may rob protein from tissues. Eating too little protein can also weaken cells.	**Protein should be about 30 percent of our calories.** Include meat in its natural form: beef, deer, goat, ox, goose, chicken, duck, quail, turkey, and fish.. **Complete Proteins** include meat, fish, poultry, cheese, eggs, milk, yogurt, and soy. **Incomplete Proteins** include grains, beans, and leafy green vegetables. **Combining foods can make a complete protein: Beans +** Brown rice, corn, nuts, seeds, or wheat **Brown Rice** + Beans, nuts, seeds, or wheat For example, add seeds or nuts to beans. Have bread with nut butter, or beans with rice in a burrito. **Omega 3 Eggs** – not only do they have protein but they also promote liver health to help the body make lecithin which breaks down fat.

Informative Notes: Signs of deficiency of protein may include failure to heal from injuries, chronic back pain, fatigue, and mood imbalances. Muscle building protein drinks can be purchased at a health food store. Some books recommend that people with fibromyalgia and arthritis should avoid red meat. "Free range" meat (from animals allowed to range and feed on grass instead of manmade feed) is always more nutritious because it has omega 3 fats (due to what the animal eats). Organic is always best because no hormones or antibiotics have been injected into the animal, or put in it's feed. Soup stock made by boiling chicken or beef with the bones acts as a digestive aid. Soup stocks made from meat cooked with the bone on it also contain cartilage and collagen which will help treat arthritis and other inflammatory conditions. Cook extra meat on the bone for supper and then reserve some stock and meat to make a soup for the next day.

Helpful Hints: Free range meat can be a little more expensive, but it may decrease your chances of becoming allergic to antibiotics or having a hormone imbalance - both of which can cost more money in the long run. **Note:** If dieting, some nutritionists advise eating protein first because it helps depress insulin secretion (insulin stores fat and prevents the breakdown of fat).

4. FATTY ACIDS / OILS (Isaiah 25:6 speaks of a feast of fat)

Genesis 45:18 says, *"...you can enjoy the fat of the land."* However, Leviticus 7:23 says, *"Do not eat any of the fat."* Leviticus is referring to the cover fat of animals which has been proven to harbor toxins. It would be impossible to avoid all marbled fat. Vegetables, seeds, and nuts have fatty acids in the form of oils which nourish our bodies. They are in abundance and are mentioned numerous times in scripture.

What God created fatty acids/oils to do for us	Eating with Purpose
Fats are composed of fatty acids which provide energy and protect internal organs. The three fatty acids needed by the body are: **Saturated** – Used by the liver to manufacture cholesterol. Some saturated fats can raise your body's level of bad cholesterol. Other saturated fats, like coconut oil, are said to be good for the heart and brain. **Polyunsaturated (Essential Fatty Acids)** - Two forms are: **Omega 3 (Alpha-linolenic) and Omega 6 (Linoleic).** EFA's lubricate your skin and tissues, reduce inflammation, flush water from kidneys, raise metabolism, and may prevent psoriasis, allergies, and diabetes. Fish oils promote heart and brain health. They may prevent neurological disorders, ADHD, Alzheimer's, and depression. You need a relatively equal ratio of omega 6 and omega 3. The typical American diet has more omega 6. A deficiency of omega 3 can lead to slow wound healing, feeling cold, joint inflammation, and repeated infections. Caution: When polyunsaturated fats are heated to a high frying temperature they turn to trans fats. **Monounsaturated Fats** – Reduces bad cholesterol while raising the good. LDL dumps excess cholesterol into arteries. HDL carries unneeded cholesterol away from cells.	**Fat should be about 30 percent of our calories.** Balancing fats can be confusing because oils can contain a mixture of different fatty acids. **Saturated (limit to 5–10%):** There is saturated fat in whole milk, cream, butter, cheese, coconut oil, and animal fat. I use mainly coconut oil for cooking. **Polyunsaturated (10-15%): Omega 3 fatty acids** include fish, fish oil, cod liver oil, walnuts, walnut oil, and omega 3 eggs. Note: Even though the yolk of an egg has cholesterol, it also has lecithin which breaks down the cholesterol. Omega 3 eggs have less saturated fat than regular eggs. **Omega 6 fatty acids** include raw nuts, seeds, legumes, vegetable oils, grape seed oil, canola oil, primrose oil, sesame oil, soybean oil, salad dressings, and flaxseed oil. Most Americans don't have to be concerned about getting enough Omega 6 fatty acids because of the amount of meat we eat. **C. Monounsaturated (10-15%):** Includes olive oil, almonds, avocados, and macadamia nuts. Olives keep insulin levels low by blocking carbohydrates

Informative Notes: Try to buy expeller/cold pressed, unrefined oil. Eliminate hydrogenated oils and fried foods. Also, some research indicates that canola oil and vegetable oils may be unstable, and can turn into trans fats.

Helpful Hints: A sign of deficiency of fatty acids can be that bowel stools do not float (fat floats). To achieve a balance of fatty acids, most Americans need to make an effort to limit saturated fats because they are in so much of our normal diet. However, coconut oil is one saturated fat that is very healthy for your brain, as well as your heart. And it actually helps you to burn other fats. Most nutritionists recommend taking fish oil. For monounsaturated fat, I use olive oil for homemade salad dressings. For cooking at high temperatures I use coconut oil.. We snack on nuts (they not only have oils, but they also have fiber, amino acids, and vitamins). Remember – no margarine or shortening.

Notes (write down your plan for eating healthy)

4 - Divine Health and Healing in...
Other Food Nutrients

Phytonutrients and Other Antioxidants Herbs, Spices, and Oils

Common Foods and their Healing Power Vitamins, Minerals, and Amino Acids

Do not be wise in your own eyes; fear the LORD and shun evil. This will bring

health to your body and nourishment to your bones.

Proverbs 3:7-8

In addition to the four basic food nutrients (macro-nutrients), God created additional nutrients (micro-nutrients) in food, which not only nourish our bodies, but also protect us from disease. This chapter covers those nutrients. It includes a variety of charts outlining healing nutrients from various perspectives.

However, due to mass production, much of our food supply has been somewhat depleted of these nutrients. Many of us don't live where we can get fresh, organic foods at a reasonable price. Therefore, many nutritionists advise taking supplements. Keep in mind however, that supplements are not meant to replace any single food source. They are meant to do just what their name implies – supplement your diet. Hopefully, that diet will be one designed according to God's plan.

Included in this chapter are several lists of foods according to the nutrients they contain, and which ailments some doctors and nutritionists feel may be alleviated by the nutrients in those foods. The lists are not intended to be used as medical advice. They are intended to inspire a well-balanced diet which includes a variety of foods. Seeing how each nutrient may contribute to overall health and healing can help to motivate us to choose healthy foods.

Two people from whom to seek advice concerning the use of supplements are a physician who believes in alternative treatments and a nutritionist at your health food store. They can often refer you to helpful resources. If you're told you need a certain supplement for a particular illness, use the following pages to determine which foods will help to supply that need as well. You may want to go through the list and circle any needs you have. Then increase the food items listed as sources for whatever nutrient you may be lacking. Take the advice of your doctor, but be willing to actively participate in your own health care by doing your own research.

Special Note: Any time you see the word *essential* on a supplement it means that the nutrient is not produced in the body, such as some amino acids. In other words, it is essential that you get it in foods, supplements, or oils applied to the skin. *Nonessential* means your body produces it so it is not essential that you find it in food. However, because of the over processing of food, you may need a normally *nonessential* supplement. Supplements can be taken in capsules, as drops under the tongue (the most powerful), or in liquid form.

PHYTO-NUTRIENTS created by God in the GOOD CARB FOODS

Phyto (or plant) nutrients are chemicals in fruits and vegetables which act as antioxidants in the body, protecting it from pollutants and free radicals. Pollutants and excess free radicals, combined with a lack of phytonutrients, can lead to cancer, macular degeneration, a rise in blood pressure, destruction of nerve cells, damaged sperm, arthritis, skin rashes, and even acne. There are thousands of phytonutrients in vegetables and fruits. Following are just a few to encourage you to eat more of these God given disease fighters. For further study of phytonutrients see *Toxic Relief* (Colbert, 2003. 113-128).

What God created phytonutrients to do for us	Foods containing phytonutrients
Carotenoids are plant pigments that don't just prevent cancer; they **fight carcinogens and guard your cells.** They prevent cancer, heart disease, and boost your immune system. Two of the main carotenoids are: **Lycopene** – a carotenoid which fights prostate and colon cancer. **Lutein** – a carotenoid for your eyes.	**Carotenoids** are in the red, orange, yellow, and dark green vegetables (carrots, watermelon, pink grapefruit, sweet potatoes, squash, tomatoes, spinach, cantaloupe, and yams). **Tomatoes interfere with chemical unions needed to create carcinogens.** Tomatoes are loaded with carotenoids. **Lycopene** is found in the red pigment of carrots, tomatoes, pink grapefruit, and watermelon. **Lutein** is found in yellow squash, corn, and spinach.
Cruciferous vegetables **detoxify** your body, thus aiding your immune system. They may also help fight breast and colon cancer.	**Cruciferous** vegetables include broccoli, sprouts, cauliflower, and radishes. **When a cancer molecule enters a cell, a nutrient in broccoli can whisk it out before it can cause harm.**
Bioflavonoids are the chemicals in plants that protect them from such things as parasites and bacteria. As we eat them, they **protect our cells from free radical damage and pollutants.** They are often called the **anti-cancer agent** in foods. They are good for younger looking skin and may help prevent heart disease. **Quercetin** is believed to fight allergies.	**Bioflavonoids** give plants their red, blue, or purple color. Blackberries, blueberries, cherries, grapes, broccoli, peppers, and tomatoes all contain bioflavonoids. **Berries keep cancer hormones from latching on to cells.** Green tea is also an excellent source. **Quercetin** is found in onions and apples.
Chlorophyll is the green pigment in plants which is believed to act as a **tumor fighter** and an anti-inflammatory agent. Two Chlorophyll phytonutrients are: **Chlorophyllin** – Cleanses the body by **removing toxins.** **Allium** – Acts as an antibacterial, anti-fungal, antiviral anti-parasitic agent. It also cleanses the body of lead and mercury.	**Chlorophyll** is found in leafy greens such as spinach, collards, parsley, alfalfa sprouts, green tea, and milk thistle. For **Chlorophyllin**, besides eating the above leafy greens, several nutritionists recommend getting a powdered "Green Superfood" from a health food store which contains wheat grass, barley grass, alfalfa, blue-green algae, green tea, grape seed extract, and milk thistle. **Allium** is found in garlic and onions. Numerous **chemicals in Garlic and onions fight carcinogens.**
Ellagic Acid helps rid the body of free radicals thus inhibiting cancer formation.	**Ellagic Acid** is found in pomegranates, raspberries, blackberries, strawberries, and grapes.
I **shop by color** and cook a minimum of two colors of vegetables at a time.	

Other antioxidants: The body's own natural antioxidant is glutathione. Its production can be stimulated by eating certain foods or taking certain supplements. The top antioxidant foods include raisins, blueberries, blackberries, garlic, and prunes and strawberries. Citrus fruits possess every class of natural substances that neutralize chemicals. Green tea is also a powerful antioxidant.

The information in the following micro-nutrient charts are brief lists that I compiled from numerous resources. *Prescription for Nutritional Healing* contains a more complete list (Balch, 2003. Part One) and can be found in most health food stores.

Antioxidant	Needed For	Food Sources
Vitamin A – Alpha-Lipoic Acid	Stimulates glutathione in the body. Helps absorb Co Q10 (see below). It is both water and fat soluble (can penetrate water and fat soluble compartments to rid them of free radicals). Helps nerves and regulates blood sugar.	Spinach, broccoli, meats, fish liver oil, bright colored fruits and vegetables.
Coenzyme Q10	Generates cellular energy, anti-aging agent, and helps heart health. Protects cells. Aids mental functions. Protects stomach lining.	Mackerel, salmon, sardines, spinach, peanuts, and beef. Can also be purchased in supplements.
Garlic	Helps rid the body of heavy metals. Protects against oxidation. Prevents fats from being oxidized. Great for the heart.	Comes fresh or in tablet form.
Ginkgo Biloba	Antioxidant for the brain. May have a positive effect against dementia and strokes. Enhances concentration and memory, and helps hearing problems.	An herb found in supplemental form. Doctors advise not taking Ginkgo Biloba with pain killers or blood thinners as the combination may result in internal bleeding.

Antioxidants (Cont.)	Needed For	Food Sources
Glutathione	This antioxidant is found in the body. It's difficult to absorb as a supplement, however, you may raise levels of it through a combination of other anitoxidants.	Taking NAC (an amino acid supplement), vitamin C, and Milk Thistle in combination may raise levels of glutathione in the body. (See Dr. Colbert's book, *Toxic Relief,* 2003. 125)
Green Tea	Acts as an antibacterial, antiviral agent. May fight cancer, cholesterol, clotting, and promote fat loss.	Found in most supermarkets. Numerous herbalists recommend drinking green tea at least twice a day.
Melatonin	Can permeate any cell in the body to rid it of free radicals. Encourages sleep.	Tablets or capsules
NAC	An amino acid which converts to glutathione (see above) in the body. Used in detoxing.	Tablets or capsules
Selenium	A trace mineral that works with vitamin E to protect tissues and cell membranes.	Garlic, asparagus, and grains (depends on the soil).
Silymarin (Milk Thistle)	Guards the liver from toxins and drugs. Promotes new liver cells. Helps increase glutathione in your body.	Milk thistle, tea, and capsules.
Vitamin C	Empowers other antioxidants. Protects the brain and spinal cord from free radicals. Protects against pollution.	Berries, citrus fruits, green vegetables, broccoli, cantaloupe, grapefruit, peas, sweet peppers, tomatoes, alfalfa, cayenne, paprika, and raspberry leaf.
Vitamin E d-alpha tocopherol Don't use dl-alpha which is synthetic	Prevents oxidation of fats. Fat soluble so it can rid fat of toxins. Improves oxygen levels. May prevent cataracts.	Leafy greens, legumes, nuts, seeds, whole grains, brown rice, cornmeal, eggs, kelp, milk, oatmeal, wheat germ, alfalfa, and raspberry leaf.
Zinc	Prevents fat oxidation. Works with vitamins A and E.	Egg yolks, fish, kelp, lamb, legumes, lima beans, meat, mushrooms, pecans, poultry, seeds, seafood, soy lecithin, sunflower seeds, alfalfa, and parsley.

Disease Fighting Powers Created by God in HERBS AND SPICES
(Use in Cooking or Drink as Teas)
Herbs contain vitamins and minerals. They also have numerous phytochemicals.

The Bible lists numerous plants and herbs which were used by the Israelites. In *The Maker's Diet*, Jordan Rubin lists what he believes are the 21 top healing herbs. They include Aloe, Black Cumin, Black Mustard, Cinnamon, Coriander, Cumin, Dandelion, Dill, Henna, Fengreek, Frankincense, Garlic, Hyssop, Juniper, Milk Thistle, Mint, Myrrh, Nettle, Saffron, Spikenard, and Turmeric (2004. 179– 186). Below are listed some common herbs readily available in the produce or baking section, and/or in teas. Some are found in supplement form. Caution: while it's safe to cook with herbs, you should consult your health care professional or a nutritionist before taking them as supplements to treat an ailment. Many come in comprehensive forms as a supplement. For instance, there is a product called *Kidney and Bladder* with seven herbs which focus on the kidney and bladder. It amazes me that God put so many healing powers in such small little leaves. These herbs contain vitamins, minerals, amino acids, and phytonutrients. Some herbs can be used as teas. Others can only be applied topically. Listed below are ways they may provide health benefits.

Aloes: An aid for burns and skin irritations. C l e a n s e s the stomach, treats teenage acne, bruises, skin inflammations, and sprains.

Alfalfa: Used to fight anemia and arthritis. Strengthens bones and joints. Aids the digestive system.

Basil: Anti-inflammatory. Cardiovascular health, protection against bacterial growth, protects cell structures.

Chamomile (Tea): Used to treat fever, heart disease, aches, pains, menstrual cramps, and stomach distress. Acts as a sleep aid. Do not use if you have allergies.

Cinnamon (Tea): Calms the stomach. Acts as an anti-tumor agent, antiseptic, anti-virus, and may prevent urinary tract infections. Add cinnamon spice to any tea, cereal, or sprinkle on toast.

Clove (Tea): Relieves nausea and vomiting, curbs gas pain, and improves digestion. Acts as a general sleep aid.

Coriander or Cilantro: Helps with acid indigestion, gas, rheumatism, toothaches, and elimination of harmful metals from the body. Contains natural chemicals that help control body odor.

Cumin: Acts as an antioxidant, disinfectant, pain reliever, and an appetite stimulant. May help with abnormal heartbeat, asthma, dermatitis, and impotence.

Dandelion (Tea): May help with anemia, cleansing the blood and liver, increasing bile, relieving menopausal symptoms, constipation, and age spots. Supports kidneys. Treats abscesses.

Dill: Helps fight cancer and estrogen deficiency. Acts as a digestive aid against gas, prevents growth of bad bacteria in the intestinal tract, relieves upper respiratory ailments, and acts as a uterine relaxant.

Echinacea (Tea): Helps against bacterial and viral infections, and stimulates white blood cells. Helps against allergies, colds, and flu. Caution: Avoid if allergic to ragweed.

Garlic: Detoxes the body, boosts immune function, lowers blood pressure, and regulates blood sugar. Helps with arthritis, asthma, cancer, colds, flu, heart, digestion, insomnia, sinusitis, and yeast infection. Fights literally any infection or disease.

Ginger (Tea): Acts as an anti-inflammatory agent. Treats cramps, bowel disorders, arthritis, hot flashes, indigestion, motion sickness, muscle pain, and nausea. Acts as an antioxidant. Can grate fresh ginger into any tea.

Ginkgo: Aids in brain function and helps memory loss. Treats headaches, leg cramps, asthma, depression, and heart disorders. Caution: Do not take with blood thinners.

Disease Fighting Powers Created by God in HERBS AND SPICES (Cont.)
Ginseng (Tea): Used to treat stress, immune system, bronchitis, circulatory problems, lack of energy and appetite.
Goldenseal (Tea): Used to fight infection and cleanse the body. Strengthens colon, liver, pancreas, spleen, and the respiratory system. Helps with allergies and bladder disorders.
Green Tea (Tea): The tea with the richest source of antioxidants. Used to fight mental fatigue, aging, cancer, cholesterol, clotting, tooth decay, and asthma. Regulates blood sugar and insulin levels.
Hyssop (Tea): A member of the mint family. Used to treat upper respiratory problems. May soothe bronchitis, flu, and asthma. A digestive aid.
Marshmallow (Tea): Expels excess mucus, heals skin and tissues, bladder infection, digestion, fluid retention, headache, kidney problems, and sinusitis.
Milk Thistle (Tea): Prevents and repairs liver damage. Lowers blood sugar and insulin levels. Has eight anti-inflammatory compounds. Can help to prevent and repair liver damage. Cleanses the liver.
Mint: May fight Alzheimer's disease. Acts as a digestive aid, and antiallergenic. Stimulates brain activity. (Mint was used on the floor of synagogues.)
Myrrh: See Healing Oils page.
Nettle (Tea): May alleviate arthritis symptoms as well as hay fever.
Parsley: May prevent multiplication of tumor cells, expels worms, relieves gas, aids digestion, freshens breath, helps bladder, kidney, liver, thyroid, stomach problems, high blood pressure, and fights obesity.
Red Raspberry (Tea): Strengthens nails, bones, teeth, and skin. Helps against menstrual bleeding, uterine spasms, diarrhea, cramps, canker sores, and morning sickness. Strengthens uterine walls.
Rosemary: Fights free radicals and bacteria. Relaxes the stomach. Acts as a decongestant. Aids in circulation to the brain. Cleanses the liver. Anticancer and anti-tumor powers. Headaches and cramps.
Sage: Aids the central nervous system. Reduces sweating, hot flashes, estrogen deficiency, and tonsillitis. Use as a hair rinse for shine and hair growth.
Saffron: The world's most expensive spice. Aids gastric problems, bladder, kidney, and liver ailments. Acts as a sedative and an expectorant.
Spikenard: Helps against epilepsy, hysteria, heart palpitations, and chorea.
Thyme (Tea): Used to treat bronchitis and phlegm. Acts as an antiseptic. A good germ killer in toothpaste.
Turmeric: Anti-inflammatory and antioxidant properties. Digestive aid, liver protector, heart tonic, and anti-arthritic properties.
Informative Notes: Ancient societies thought herbs contained spirits because they would be healed of diseases when they ate them. The healing properties were true, but what they worshiped was really a chemical. These chemicals were placed in herbs by God. The Israelites used herbs to season food and in the treatment of illness. (Read Song of Solomon 4:13-15)
Helpful Hints: (1/2 teaspoon dried = 1 Tablespoon fresh). I began by using one herb at a time. I alternate an all-purpose herb seasoning with Italian Seasoning (on zucchini, tomatoes and onions all sautéed together). If I'm not sure about the taste, I sprinkle the herbs on a small portion in the pan and taste it. If I like it, I put it on the rest of the food. I freeze fresh herbs wrapped in a paper towel and placed in a freezer bag. Just before cooking, I chop off what I need and put the rest back in the freezer. Note: I have included several salad dressing recipes using a variety of herbs (see Chapter 6).

Topical Essential Oils God Gave us for Health and Healing

While not all of these are food items, they can be applied externally. Check with your health food store to see which oils would be best to suit your needs and how they should be applied. Some are very powerful and must be mixed with oil.

They may seem expensive but they last a long time. You only need a few drops at a time. Start by choosing just one or two that fit your need, and then branch out to using a variety.

Some of this list is compiled from Jordan Rubin's book *The Maker's Diet,* (2004. 186-190)

The Bible mentions over 30 essential oils. Esther treated herself for 6 months with oil of Myrrh before presenting herself to the King (Esther 2:12). I put a few drops in my makeup.

Myrrh: Protects against infection, aids oral hygiene, balances thyroid, heals fungal and viral infections, and supports the immune system.

Frankincense: Helps maintain normal cellular regeneration, stimulates the immune system, aids those suffering from depression, bronchitis, and allergies.

Cedar wood: Disinfectant, hygiene, skin problems, hair loss, bronchitis, and skin disorders such as acne.

Cinnamon: Antibacterial, antiviral, boosts immune system against colds and flu.

Galbanum: Acne, asthma, coughs, indigestion, muscle aches and pains, wrinkles, and wounds.

Onycha: Soothes skin irritations, treats colic, constipation, blood sugar levels, bronchitis, colds, coughs, and sore throats.

Hyssop: Relieves anxiety, arthritis, asthma, respiratory infections, fungal infections, colds, and flu. Used to treat wounds and cuts. Metabolizes fat. Helps cleanse the body of parasites.

Sandalwood: Enhances sleep. Aids in relief of urinary traction infection.

Myrtle: Balances hormones, soothes the respiratory system, battles colds, flu, bronchitis, and coughs.

These are just a few of the oils mentioned in Rubin's book. They are very high in their antioxidant capacity. He says that one ounce of clove oil has the antioxidant capacity of 450 pounds of carrots (2004. 186).

Most oils can be found in small bottles in your health food store or at shops like Bath and Body. I keep a mixture of 12 drops of Frankincense, plus 12 drops of Myrrh (mixed in 1.5 ounces of olive oil) on hand. I pray as I apply it to an area of need. I figure that if these were given to Jesus by Kings they must be good for many things. I personally experienced relief from inflammation through application to my back and knees. Oils can also be put in shampoos, hand lotions, or in your bath.

Some symptoms (such as Athlete's Foot) may require that you take some form of supplement internally, as well as apply a natural ointment externally. That way you're fighting the fungus both ways.

For a more in-depth study concerning the healing power of herbs, read the following scriptures about the use of hyssop and cedar wood: Exodus 12:22, Leviticus 14:4, Numbers 19:18, Psalms 51:7, John 19:29 and Hebrews 9:19. God uses Hyssop as a physical symbol to reveal a spiritual truth because there are physical healing and cleansing properties in Hyssop that reveal the truth of spiritual healing and cleansing.

Your name is like anointing oil poured out. Hebrews 1:9

Disease Fighting Powers That God Placed in Common Foods: The next three pages list food items and the healing nutrients God created in them. Isaiah advised King Hezekiah to treat his boils with a poultice of figs and he recovered (2 Kings 20:7).

Apples	Reduces cholesterol. Contains anti-cancer agents. Antibacterial, antiviral, anti-inflammatory properties. Estrogenic activity. Contains fiber. Suppresses the appetite.
Asparagus	Super source of glutathione, the body's natural antioxidant.
Avocados	Helps clear arteries by lowering bad cholesterol. Dilates blood vessels. Acts as an antioxidant. Contains glutathione. Blocks many carcinogens.
Bananas	Soothes the stomach. Strengthens stomach lining. Acts as an antibiotic. High in potassium.
Barley	Helps with heart ailments by reducing cholesterol. Antiviral, anticancer, and antioxidant.
Beans	Help lower cholesterol. Regulates blood sugar. High fiber.
Bell Peppers	Super rich antioxidant with vitamin C. Fights off colds, asthma, bronchitis, respiratory infections, cataracts, anginas, and cancer.
Blueberries	Acts as an antibiotic by blocking the attachment of bacteria to the urinary tract. Curbs diarrhea. Antioxidant, anti-viral, and a natural aspirin.
Broccoli	A versatile disease fighter. Contains numerous antioxidants such as quercetin (for allergies) glutathione, beta carotene, C, and lutein. Extremely high anticancer powers. Speeds up removal of estrogen from the body. Rich in fiber. Regulates blood sugar.
Cabbage	Numerous anticancer and antioxidant compounds. Speeds up estrogen metabolism. Suppresses growth of polyps. Fights colon cancer. Anti-viral agent.
Carrots	The super food for beta carotene. Anticancer, artery-protecting, immune-boosting, infection-fighting antioxidant. High in soluble fiber. Reduces odds of degenerative eye disease. Cooking does not destroy beta-carotene.
Cauliflower	Cancer-fighting and hormone-regulating activities. A cousin to broccoli and cabbage. Wards off breast and colon cancer. Heavy cooking destroys some activity. Eat raw or lightly cooked.
Celery	Aids against high blood pressure. Anticancer compounds. Detoxifies carcinogens.
Chili Peppers	Dissolves blood-clots. Opens sinuses by breaking up mucus. Expectorant.
Chocolate	Counteracts lactose intolerance. Antioxidant.
Cinnamon	Stimulates insulin activity.
Cloves	Relieves the pain of a toothache. Anti-inflammatory against rheumatic disease.
Corn	Anticancer and anti-viral properties. However, it is difficult to digest. Do not eat while preparing to cleanse (see Chapter 5).
Cranberries	Antibiotic for preventing infections. Keeps bacteria from sticking to cells.
Fish and Fish oils	Intervenes in heart disease. An ounce a day may cut the risk of heart attacks. Helps treat rheumatoid arthritis, asthma, psoriasis, migraine headaches, Multiple Sclerosis, strokes, and cancer. Cod liver oil is highly recommended.

Disease Fighting Powers That God Placed in Common Foods (Cont.)	
Garlic	Used to treat a variety of ills. Combats bacteria, intestinal parasites and viruses. Helps lower blood pressure and cholesterol: Anticancer compounds and antioxidants. Tops National Cancer Institute list as potential cancer-preventive food. Relieves gas, diarrhea, lifts moods, and has a calming effect.
Ginger	Treats nausea, vomiting, migraine headaches, chest congestion, colds, diarrhea, stomachache, and nervous diseases. Anti-ulcer, anti-depressant, anticancer agent. Treats cramps.
Grapes	Rich in antioxidants. Antibacterial, anti-viral, and anticancer agent.
Grapefruit	The pulp contains a unique pectin that lowers blood cholesterol and reverses clogged arteries. Anti-cancer (stomach and pancreas). High vitamin C.
Honey	Contains enzymes, minerals, amino acids and vitamins. Antibiotic, sleep inducing and tranquilizing.
Kiwi	Aids against stomach and breast cancer. Vitamin C.
Licorice	Strong anticancer agents. Kills bacteria. (Too much can raise blood pressure.)
Melon	Anticoagulant activity. Contains the antioxidant beta carotene.
Milk	Cancer fighter in the colon, lungs, stomach, and cervix. (Can trigger allergic reactions.)
Mushrooms	Heart medicine, and cancer remedy. Treats viral diseases, and influenza. May cut cholesterol. Shitake mushrooms may fight leukemia. There is little value in button mushrooms.
Mustard	Decongestant. Breaks up mucus. Antibacterial. Revs up metabolism by 25 percent, burning off extra calories.
Nuts	Anticancer and heart preventative powers. Walnuts are a cancer fighter. Almonds reduce cholesterol with antioxidant properties. Brazil nuts are extremely rich in selenium – an antioxidant against heart disease and cancer. Walnuts are high in omega 3. Nuts, seeds, and grains all have enzymes which aid digestion. However they also have enzymes inhibitors placed in them by God to protect them from harmful substances. It's best to soak them to release these enzyme inhibitors (or take an enzyme supplement).
Oats	Depresses cholesterol. Stabilizes blood sugar. Antioxidant. Fiber.
Olive Oil	An artery protector that lowers bad LDL. Regulates blood sugar. Antioxidant and anticancer.
Onion, shallots, chives,	One of the oldest medicines. Thought to cure about everything – strong antioxidant. Numerous anticancer agents. Thins blood, lowers bad cholesterol. Fights asthma, bronchitis, and hay fever. Acts as a sedative.
Oranges	Complete package of natural cancer inhibitors. Rich in vitamin C and beta carotene. Fights pancreatic cancer, asthma, bronchitis, and gum disease. Boosts fertility. Citrus Fruits have 58 known anticancer chemicals.
Parsley	High concentration of numerous antioxidants. Anticancer – detoxifies carcinogens and neutralizes tobacco smoke.
Pineapple	Suppresses inflammation. Contains antibacterial enzymes. Aids digestion. Good for the bones. The core of a pineapple is high in the enzyme bromelain for aid in digestion.

Disease Fighting Powers That God Placed in Common Foods (Cont.)	
Plums/ Prunes	High antioxidant. Laxative. Antibacterial and anti-viral properties. Prunes are a natural aspirin.
Potatoes	High in potassium. Some estrogenic activity.
Pumpkin	Extremely high in beta carotene.
Raspberries	Anti-viral, anticancer. Natural aspirin. Red raspberry tea – regulates menstrual cramps and flow.
Rice	Anti-diarrhea. Anticancer. Least likely to cause gas as a fiber. Can soothe upset stomach.
Spinach	Tops the list along with other leafy greens as the food most eaten by people who don't get cancer. Super antioxidant. High in beta carotene and lutein. Rich in fiber. Lowers cholesterol. Not recommended for people with kidney stones.
Strawberries	Anti-viral, anticancer agent for overall types of cancer. This is the one fruit that you should definitely buy organic. It is porous and cannot be adequately rinsed.
Sweet potatoes	High in the antioxidant beta carotene. Prevents heart disease, cataracts, strokes, and numerous cancers.
Tea (herbal)	Anticoagulant, artery protector, antibiotic, anti-ulcer, cavity-fighter, antidiarrheal, antiviral, and analgesic. Green Tea helps block skin cancers, stomach cancers, and lung cancers. Asian Green Tea is best. Black tea is not as effective.
Tomatoes	Major source of lycopene – antioxidant and anticancer agents that intervene with the chain reaction of oxygen free radical molecules. Prevents pancreatic and cervical cancer.
Vinegar	Bragg's is a good brand. Helps maintain a healthy pH balance. Helps you to lose weight. Keeps you hydrated. My health coach drinks 1 –2 teaspoons of Bragg's vinegar, with 1 – 2 teaspoons of pure honey, stirred into 8 ounces of water for overall health and weight management.
Watermelon	High amounts of lycopene and glutathione. Acts as an antioxidant and anticancer agent.
Wheat	High fiber. Ranks as the world's greatest preventatives of constipation and therefore anticancer agent. Can suppress polyps. Some doctors say white flour can contribute to rheumatoid arthritis symptoms.
Yogurt	Antibacterial and anticancer properties. A cup a day boosts immune functioning by attacking viruses. Prevents and cures diarrhea. Prevents yeast infection with acidophilus. Contains calcium for strong bones. Fermented foods, like yogurt, contain live cultures. They are good to eat before and after fasting to replace any good bacteria lost in the intestines. Kefir (now in most supermarkets) is like a liquid yogurt. The taste can be improved by blending in fresh or frozen berries. Fermented foods also help with mental alertness.

Health Notes: Our God is a loving and caring God that gave us food, not just to fill our stomachs, but to keep us in health. This information freed me from thinking God's food laws were a restrictive burden. The opposite is true: God gave us food to free us from disease. Thanking God for our food at meal time has taken on new meaning for us. If you are suffering from a chronic disorder, make a list of the foods which contain the nutrients God gave us for the healing of that disease. Again, do some research on your own and be an active participant in experiencing the healing God has promised His children. For more information on the healing power of food, read *What the Bible Says About Healthy Living*, by Dr. Rex Russell.

Symptoms and Illnesses Which May be Alleviated by the Healing Power of Common Foods

This list is arranged by the illness first, followed by a list of foods which may prevent and even sometimes reverse that illness. It is not intended as medical advice, but merely to stimulate your interest in looking to nutrition in addition to conventional treatments. For more specific information on treating illnesses through alternative methods read *Prescription for Nutritional Healing* (Balch, 2000. Part Two*)*. It is like an encyclopedia of common ailments and suggestions for treatment. You might also consider doing your own research by typing the name of the disease in a search engine on the internet. Keep in mind, there is some very unwise advice on the internet, as well as what is viable. Do some research at your library as well.

Become an active participant in your health care, but discuss your findings with your doctor and a health food consultant. (Note: My health coach advised me that viruses, bacteria, and cancer feed on sugar)

Symptoms	Foods which may help alleviate symptoms
Acne	High fiber diet, fish, lots of fruits, sunflower seeds. Zinc is an antibacterial agent. Drink 8 glasses of water a day. Avoid caffeine and dairy. Go to Proactiv.com for a topical treatment. Evening primrose oil is good for the complexion.
Allergies	Peppers, white part of the orange under the peel, grapes. Lessen or eliminate milk and sugars. Focus on foods that have bioflavonoids (page 16) like onions and grapes. Plain yogurt with thawed berries stirred in.
Arthritis	Fish, cod liver oil, fresh vegetables, and ginger. No sugar. Some doctors advise avoiding wheat and milk for a while as well. Read *Arthritis for Dummies*.
Asthma	Onions, garlic, fish, fruits and vegetables are anti-inflammatory agents. Hot peppers and spicy food clear air passages. Avoid vegetable oils.
Bladder Infection	Cranberries and blueberries. Prevents bacteria from sticking to cells of the urinary tract. Avoid caffeine and chocolate.
Brain Power Food Brain Power Diet	Protein, seafood, skim-milk, and tea. Downers – sugar, pastas, bread, and fat. Breakfast: Skim milk, fruit, hard-boiled egg, Ezekiel bread, herbal tea. Lunch: Plain tuna, chicken, or turkey. Green salad, fresh vegetables, fruit, and low fat cottage cheese. Dinner: Broiled fish, green vegetables, tomatoes, and berries. No desserts. No junk food. No starchy foods. No high fat foods.
Breast Cancer	Cabbage, broccoli, vitamin C, fruits and vegetables, fish, and wheat bran. Avoid fatty red meat. No hydrogenated fat.
Calorie-Burners	Hot spicy foods speed up metabolism as do mustard and ginger. Mustard increases metabolism by 25 percent. Weight loss – Lecithin breaks down fat.
Cholesterol	See chapter 5 about cleansing. Coconut oil, salmon, garlic cloves, oats, onions, olive oil, almonds, walnuts, avocados, strawberries, broccoli, apples, carrots, and grapefruit. Eat a wide variety of beans, fruits, and vegetables.
Colds	Chicken soup, spicy foods, vitamin C, garlic, thyme, and rosemary. Echinacea and Goldenseal tea if not allergic to rag weed. Three months before pollen season, eat yogurt. Focus on foods with bioflavonoids.
Colon Cancer	All Bran, Wheat Bran and Oat Cereals. Seafood, green vegetables, and dried beans. Beta carotenes may fight cancer and destroy tumor cells. Garlic, onions, cabbage, broccoli, radishes, tomatoes, and green tea are enemies of carcinogens. Oranges may neutralize carcinogens. Reduce fatty red meats and eat no hydrogenated fats. Special Note: Cancer may feed on sugar. For more information go to cancernutrition.com.

Symptoms and Illnesses Which May be Alleviated Through the Healing Power of Foods (Cont.)	
Symptom	**Food which may help alleviate symptoms**
Constipation	Water, coarse wheat bran, flaxseed oil, rice bran, fruits, vegetables, prunes, and vitamin C. Exercise.
Depression	Fish, raw fruits and vegetables, whole grains, seeds, nuts, and brown rice. Spinach, seafood, carbohydrates, caffeine, garlic, tuna and nuts are all mood lifters. Avoid junk food, sugar, and white flour.
Diabetes	Beans, high fiber, high carb, starch, pasta, rice, and oats.
Diarrhea / Upset Stomach	Starchy soups, plain yogurt, rice, and root vegetables. Avoid milk, fruit juices, coffee, beans, fruit and vegetable peels, high sugar drinks, coffee, and diet candies. Eat 1/2 cup of cooked rice. Drink ginger and peppermint teas. Avoid roughage, fried foods, salted foods, cabbage, and citrus juices.
Gas	The most common cause is a lack of enzymes to digest beans, milk, sugar, oat bran, starch, broccoli, and cabbage. Many nutritionists are now recommending taking enzyme supplements. Ginger tea helps gas. Rinse beans twice when cooking. Add garlic to food.
Headaches	Feverfew herb. Fish, fish oil, and ginger. Avoid triggers: chocolate, caffeine, msg, aspartame, cured meats, aged cheese, nuts, alcohol, ice cream, raisins, and hot dogs.
Heartburn	The top cause is a sluggish digestive tract which causes a reaction to chocolate, fats, peppermint, garlic, onion, orange juice, hot sauce, tomatoes, and coffee. They relax the sphincter muscle allowing stomach acid to back up into the esophagus. Don't lie down for 3 hours after eating – lie on left side. Consider doing a cleanse (see chapter 5).
Heart Trouble	Fish – Omega 3 fatty acids block blood platelets, reduce blood vessel constriction, increase blood flow, block cell damage, raise good HDL, and make membranes more flexible. Garlic can reverse the damage by healing arteries. Eat a few raw nuts every day. Fruits and vegetables help keep arteries unclogged. Cook with olive oil. Eliminate all trans fats. Read *Maximum Energy* by Ted Broer.
Immunity	Green Tea, shitake mushrooms, garlic, beta carotene, vegetables, fruits, and fish.
Kidney Stones	Fruits, vegetables, high fiber grains, and water. Avoid high protein diets, sodium, overuse of spin- ach, rhubarb, and peanuts. Drink fresh squeezed lemon juice routinely.
Menopause	Black Cohash and Red Clover herbs in tablet form. Progesterone cream (not estrogen).
Menstrual Problems	Limit caffeine and sugar. Ginger and peppermint tea. Eat 5 small meals with plenty of fresh fruits and vegetables. Drink plenty of water. Before going to bed eat small portions of oats, potatoes, or bread.

These notes are just brief listings from suggested alternative treatments by the nutritionists and doctors I read. Again, they are not a cure all. Unfortunately, there can come a point where it's too late to rely on food and supplements for healing. But don't give up hope. Jordan Rubin, in *The Maker's Diet*, tells how he was healed of Crohn's disease through alternative treatments – after 70 doctors in 12 countries were unable to help him. If you have a chronic disorder, I would suggest that you read his book for inspiration and help. Another easy to understand book is *Maximum Energy* by Ted Broer.

Vitamins, Minerals, and Amino Acids – Other than a multivitamin, many nutritionists suggest getting most of your individual vitamins from your diet, unless you have a special need or sign of deficiency. For example, most women need a B-Complex. The amount should be adjusted according to body size, activities, stress level, ailments, medications, and diet. (Note: Be sure to read labels when taking vitamins. A, D, E, and K are fat soluble so they must be taken with food.) *Prescription for Nutritional Healing*, by Phyllis Balch CNC and James F. Balch, M.D., contains lists of common illnesses along with recommended supplementation programs (2000. Part One).

Vitamin:	Needed for	Food Sources
A	Eyes, skin, immunity, ulcers, epithelial tissue, bones, teeth, fat storage, colds, flu, diseases, bladder, lungs, antioxidant, new cell growth, heart disease, and aging.	Green and yellow fruits and vegetables: broccoli, cantaloupe, carrots, garlic, peaches, pumpkin, red peppers, spinach, sweet potatoes, watercress, parsley, and paprika, alfalfa, raspberry leaves, and sage. Animal sources are liver, and fish oils.
B1 Thiamin	Nerves, skin, eyes, hair, liver, mouth, muscle tone, gastrointestinal tract, brain function, circulation, blood formation, cognitive activity, energy.	Brown rice, egg yolks, fish, legumes, liver, peanuts, peas, pork, poultry, rice bran, wheat germ, whole grains, oatmeal, dried prunes, raisins, alfalfa, parsley, cayenne, and sage.
B2 Riboflavin	Red blood cell formation, eye fatigue, cataracts, metabolism, digestive tract, oxygen, hair loss, insomnia, and slowed mental response.	Cheese, egg yolks, fish, legumes, meat, milk, poultry, spinach, whole grains. Broccoli, avocados, leafy greens, nuts, watercress, alfalfa, parsley, peppermint, raspberry leaves, cayenne, and sage.
B3 Niacinamide	Circulation, healthy skin, nervous system, hydrochloric acid, and sex hormones.	Beef liver, broccoli, carrots, cheese, corn flour, dates, eggs, fish, milk, peanuts, pork, potatoes, tomatoes, wheat germ, cayenne, pars- ley, raspberry leaf, and alfalfa.
B 5 Pantothenic Acid	Anti-stress vitamin. Helps with adrenal hormones, antibodies, anemia, anxiety, and depression. Aids vitamin utilization.	Beef, eggs, fresh vegetables, kidney, legumes, liver, nuts, saltwater fish, whole rye flour, and wheat flour.
B6	Aids more body functions than any other nutrient: physical and mental. Cell formation, nervous system, synthesis, reproduction of all cells, immune system, head-aches, and fatigue.	Carrots, eggs, fish, meat, peas, spinach, sunflower seeds, walnuts, wheat germ, avocado, bananas, beans, broccoli, brown rice, whole grains, cantaloupe, corn, potatoes, rice bran, and alfalfa.
B12 (Needed to synthesize other B vitamins)	Spinal cord degeneration, learning ability, memory, migraines, heart palpitations, anemia, digestion, fertility, growth, nerve endings, bone loss, dizziness, and ringing in ears.	Eggs, herring, liver, kidney, mackerel, milk, dairy, seafood, and alfalfa.

Vitamin	Needed for	Food Sources
Biotin	Cell growth, fatty acid, metabolism, and hair loss.	Egg yolks, meat, milk, poultry, saltwater fish, soybeans, and whole grains.
Choline	Nerve impulse transmission, gallbladder, liver, lecithin formation, and hormones.	Egg yolks, lecithin, legumes, meat, milk, soybeans, and whole grain cereals.
Folic Acid (folate)	Brain food, energy, formation of blood cells, and protein metabolism.	Asparagus, barley, beef, bran, brown rice, cheese, chicken, green leafy veggies, legumes, milk, peas, pork, root veggies, salmon, tuna, wheat germ, and whole grains.
Inositol	Hair growth, irritability, skin eruptions, calms nerves, reduces cholesterol, pre- vents hardening of arteries, helps in formation of lecithin, metabolizes fat and cholesterol. Removes fat from liver.	Fruit, lecithin, legumes, meats, milk, molasses, raisins, vegetables, and whole grains.
PABA	Assimilates pantothenic acid. Antioxidant, skin cancer, red blood cells, and intestinal flora.	Kidney, liver, spinach, and whole grains.
C Ester	Raises glutathione antioxidant, tissue, gums, anti-stress, immune system, asthma, pollution, cancer, infection, bones, collagen, and cartilage.	Berries, citrus fruits, green vegetables, broccoli, cantaloupe, grapefruit, peas, sweet peppers, tomatoes, alfalfa, cayenne, paprika, and raspberry leaf.
Bioflavonoids (mixed) Rutin (Quecertin) Hesperidin	Absorption of C. Allergies. Relieves pain, bumps, bruises, capillaries, antibacterial, lowers cholesterol, cataracts, and asthma. Quercetin – Allergies such as allergic rhinitis. Inhibits release of histamine.	Grapes, berries, apples, garlic, tomatoes, broccoli, milk thistle (silymarin), green tea, peppers, citrus fruits (white part), blackberries, grapefruit, grapes, and lemons.Onions, apples, and broccoli have quercetin for allergies.
D3	Helps with absorption of calcium for bones, teeth, and muscles. Helps heartbeat, thyroid, and fight against cancer.	Fish liver oils, saltwater fish, dairy, eggs, butter, egg yolks, halibut, liver, milk, oatmeal, salmon, sweet potatoes, tuna, alfalfa, and parsley. The sun is a good source.
E d-alpha-tocopherol	Cancer, heart, circulation, tissue repair, PMS, clotting, healing, blood pressure, leg cramps, and skin.	Vegetable oils, green leafy veggies, legumes, nuts, seeds, whole grains, brown rice, cornmeal, eggs, kelp, milk, oatmeal, wheat germ, alfalfa, and raspberry leaf.
K	Used to clot blood. Needed for bones, and liver.	Asparagus, broccoli, leafy greens, egg yolks, oatmeal, oats, rye, wheat, alfalfa, and green tea.

Mineral	Needed for	Food Sources
Boron **Picolinate or citrate**	Bones, muscles, metabolism of other minerals, alertness, and energy. Helps the body use calcium.	Apples, carrots, grapes, leafy greens, nuts, pears, and whole grains.
Calcium	Strong bones and teeth, heartbeat. Reduces cramps. (Must be taken with magnesium for absorption.)	Dairy, salmon, seafood, leafy greens, almonds, asparagus, broccoli, buttermilk, alfalfa, cayenne, parsley, peppermint, raspberry, nuts, and seeds.
Chromium	Energy, synthesis of fats, cholesterol, proteins, blood sugar levels, anxiety, and fatigue. Most diets are deficient.	Brown rice, cheese, meat, and whole grains.
Copper Too much can damage eye tissue.	Bone, red blood cells, skin, energy, taste, and anemia	Almonds, avocados, barley, beans, broccoli, garlic, nuts, oats, oranges, pecans, raisins, salmon, seafood, soybeans, and leafy greens.
Iodine	Softens stools. Nourishes brain tis- sue, nerves, nails, and spinal cord. Prevents hair loss.	Seaweed, iodized salt, salt-water fish, onion, and milk products.
Iron	Oxygenation, immune system, energy, anemia, hair, and fatigue.	Eggs, fish, meat, poultry, leafy greens, whole grains, breads, cereals, almonds, avocados, beans, peaches, and pears.
Magnesium	Energy. Fights depression and muscle weakness. Stress. Alleviates PMS and painful joints.	Most foods. Fish, meat, seafood, apples, bananas, garlic, leafy greens, beans, nuts, and parsley. Coffee, sugar, soda pop, tobacco, and a high carb diet may cause a magnesium depletion.

Mineral	Needed for	Food Sources
Manganese	Protein and fat metabolism, nerves, immune system, blood sugar regulation, bone growth, cartilage, and joints.	Avocados, nuts, seeds, seaweed, whole grains, blueberries, egg yolks, legumes, peas, leafy greens, peppermint, and parsley.
Molybdenum	Metabolism. Cell function. Enzyme activation.	Beans, beef liver, cereal, grains, dark greens, legumes, and peas.
Potassium (citrate)	Nervous system, heart rhythm, stroke, muscle contraction, and water balance.	Bananas, dairy foods, fish, fruit, legumes, meat, poultry, vegetables, whole grains, apricots, avocados, lima beans, brown rice, garlic, nuts, potatoes, dried fruit, raisins, spinach, and wheat bran.
Selenium	Vital antioxidant, protects immune system, prevents formation of free radicals. Thyroid, tumors, and antibodies.	Meat, grains, brazil nuts, broccoli, brown rice, chicken, dairy, garlic, kelp, molasses, onions, salmon, seafood, tuna, vegetables, wheat grass, peppers, alfalfa, and parsley.
Vanadium	Cellular metabolism, bones, teeth, cholesterol, insulin, kidney disease, and impaired reproduction.	Dill, fish, olives, meat, radishes, snap beans, vegetable oils, and whole grains.
Zinc (do not take over 100 mg)	Prostate gland, reproductive organs, acne (oil glands) collagen, immune system, and healing. Fights free radicals.	Egg yolks, fish, kelp, lamb, legumes, lima beans, meat, mushrooms, pecans, poultry, seeds, seafood, soy lecithin, sunflower seeds, alfalfa, and parsley.

Amino Acids: Dietary protein is broken down into amino acids which build proteins in tissues and muscles. A variety of amino acids is needed because they work together: Too much meat causes too many amino acids and can become toxic. That's why meat-only diets can be dangerous. The list below contains only the essential amino acids which are not produced by the body and must be obtained from food sources. Some physicians advise that you should refrain from taking amino acid supplements unless directed by your health care professional. However, they advise that supplementation may be needed in cases where there is a deficiency.

Amino Acid	Needed For	Food Sources
Histidine	Growth and repair of tissues. Protects nerve cells. Too much can lead to stress, rheumatoid arthritis, and nerve deafness.	Rice, wheat, and rye.
Isoleucine	Stabilizes blood sugar. Enhances energy and endurance for athletes. Aids in healing and repair of muscles and tissue.	Almonds, cashews, chicken, eggs, fish, rye, and seeds.
Leucine	Protects muscles. Promotes healing. Increases hormone production.	Rice, beans, meat, nuts, and whole wheat.
Lysine	Growth and bone development in children. Aids in production of antibodies and hormones. Helps with collagen formation and tissue repair. Fights herpes virus, anemia, hair loss, inability to concentrate, irritability, lack of energy, and weight loss.	Cheese, eggs, fish, lima beans, milk, potatoes, red meat, and yeast.
Methionine	Breaks down fats. Helps body to detoxify heavy metals from the body. Prevents brittle hair. Treats rheumatic fever. Promotes excretion of estrogen. Reduces histamine to help with schizophrenia. Good for the brain and nerves.	Beans, eggs, fish, garlic, meat, onions, seeds, and yogurt.
Phenylalanine	May have a direct effect on brain chemistry. May elevate moods, aid in memory and learning (ADD). Suppress the appetite. Used to treat arthritis, back pain, depression, and menstrual cramps.	Meat, fish, eggs, and dairy products.
Threonine	Formation of collagen, tooth enamel. Helps prevent fatty buildup. Enhances the immune system. May aid against mental Illness and depression.	Dairy, beef, poultry, eggs, beans, nuts and seeds.
Tryptophan	Helps the brain transfer nerve impulses from one cell to another. Aids in sleep. May alleviate hyperactivity. Reduces appetite, migraine headaches, and coronary artery spasms.	Brown rice, cottage cheese, meat, and peanuts.
Valine	Muscle metabolism. Treats liver and gallbladder diseases.	Dairy, grains, meat, mushrooms, and peanuts.

Notes (write down your plan for eating healthy)

5 - Restoring Your Digestive Health

When we consistently eat an unhealthy diet, the inside of our digestive system can end up looking like a garbage dump of toxins. Sorry for the expression, but it's the best way I've heard it described. A clogged digestive system prevents nutrients from being absorbed and toxins from being released. The good news is, the body has a tremendous ability to cleanse itself – if we treat it right.

This chapter is about two very important keys to our health:

1. How we can cleanse our bodies of toxins that are already there, and

2. How we can eat healthy to increase the nutrients going into our bodies, as well as reduce additional toxins.

Both of these goals are for the purpose of living in health as God intended. Some of the doctors I read are beginning to see physical disorders completely reversed by having their patients cleanse their bodies (often referred to as detoxing). However, always remember, the body is only temporary, but the spirit is eternal. Just as food nourishes our body, the Word of God nourishes our spirit. And the truth is, our spirit has an effect on our body. No health habit will ever replace the discipline of spending time in prayer and reading God's Word. In doing so, your physical body will benefit.

Dear friend, I pray that you may enjoy good health and that all may go well with you,

even as your soul is getting along well.

3 John 2

Just as the healing qualities of food make known the truth that our God is the healer, so the parallels of spiritual and physical cleansing are fascinating. When you do a spiritual fast, your spirit is cleansed. At the same time, your body is being cleansed of toxins. Until I did this research, I was not aware of this parallel.

That doesn't mean we should stop seeking God for miraculous healing. God miraculously healed me of a foot injury. But he has also healed me through cleansing and eating the way He says to eat. After just four months of eating the way described in this chapter, I lost 14 pounds, I quit taking aspirin nearly every day for headaches, and my allergies are 95 percent gone. My husband lost 35 pounds and no longer has symptoms of acid-reflux. To me, this is just as much a divine (Godlike) healing as an instant miracle.

As you're reading the next two chapters, remember the information must be adjusted to meet your own medical concerns. This is merely a diet which we have learned is both Biblical and, what Dr. Colbert calls "liver friendly." In *Toxic Relief* he says that, before cleansing, it's important to eat healthy for two weeks in order to rest your liver (the major detoxification organ in your digestive tract). Cleansing will have little affect if it's not supported by a healthy diet. You have already listed some goals on your "My Plan" sheet for eating healthier.

After reading this chapter, write down on your "Notes" page and "My Plan" sheet which cleanse you may want to use (consult with your health care professional, but keep in mind that not all doctors are familiar with the benefits of cleansing). Once you have a handle on a healthy diet, set aside a four to five week period to focus on ridding your body of toxins. That involves following three simple steps:

1. Eat a healthy diet that is easy to digest (for two weeks).

2. Cleanse your body by using one of the plans mentioned later in this book.

3. Continue to eat a healthy diet for two more weeks. Hopefully, you will stick close to this way of eating even after cleansing. We found that our tastes changed, and we began liking the taste of many things we had not previously included in our diet.

WHERE TO BEGIN

Before eating, I asked myself:

1. Did God create this for food?
2. Has this food been artificially altered by man?
3. Am I making this food my god?

THINGS TO CONSIDER:

* We have found that observing point number two is the most difficult in today's society. For instance, when going to someone's house for dinner, it's often necessary to make a compromise. It's also necessary to consider cost. Remember, these three points are advice from a doctor, not doctrines from the Bible. We simply began with the goal of reducing toxins and increasing nutrients.
* Keep it simple at first – I've included 7 days of recipes. By the end of the 7 days, you'll have a handle on how to cook healthy. For more recipes get the *What Would Jesus Eat Cook Book* by Don Colbert, M.D.
* Don't see meat as the mainstay on your plate. While cleansing, have smaller portions of red meat.
* Do away with the American ideal of potatoes with every meal. Think rice and whole grains.
* Think 50 percent raw and 50 percent cooked vegetables. View them, along with a salad and grains, as the focus of your meal. Eat a variety and remember, the brighter the color the greater the nutrients.
* Use snack time for including fresh fruit and nuts.
* Review the nutritional benefits of one food per day to motivate yourself.
* Educate your family. Explain what God put in the food.
* Avoid white sugar and white flour (along with processed foods). Limit potatoes.
* Eliminate foods containing hydrogenated oils.
* In the last chapter (which includes a menu), I've included a snack in addition to lunch. If you're trying to lose weight you may want to choose between the snack and the lunch.
* After you have completely cleansed, begin to explore more recipes using the guidelines in this book.
* Food isn't the only cure. Exercise excretes toxins through the skin. Deep breathing cleanses your respiratory system, and using the right lotions prevents toxins from getting into your system through the skin. It's also important to consider your family history when adjusting eating habits.
* Eat slowly and chew the food well to release digestive enzymes. Don't overeat, or under-eat. Let your body tell you when it's hungry. You'll be amazed at the amount of food you can have on your plate when that food is healthier and contains fewer calories. Also, as your body cleanses itself, you'll have fewer cravings.
* Drink 16 ounces of filtered water 30 minutes before breakfast and in between every meal.
* Don't eat when you're upset. Your digestive juices are suppressed and food won't be digested properly.
* When dieting, don't eat sweets and starches on the same day. (No sweets while cleansing.)
* Shop around the outside edge of the grocery store first – where everything is fresh or frozen.

TIPS FOR EATING OUT:

* Order a double portion of vegetables, or wild rice, in place of a potato.
* Order water with no ice and include squeezed lemon juice. Lemon helps in cleansing while eating.
* Drink no more than 4 - 8 ounces of water (no ice) with your meal. It dilutes the digestive juices. Cold water slows down digestion.
* Ask if they have fresh parsley for your salad.
* Order salad dressing on the side. Ask if they have extra virgin olive oil – dilute your favorite salad dressing with olive oil. No fried foods unless it's cooked in coconut oil.

68

A Brief Review: Easy to Follow Basic Food Guide

(Print and hang this guide up in your kitchen pantry. Be sure to take your own health concerns into consideration.)

Vegetables – Buy a variety of fresh or frozen. Eat 50 percent raw and 50 percent cooked. Lightly steam or sauté in coconut or olive oil. Add some fresh garlic. If using frozen buy individual vegetables, take a handful out of the bag and toss them in the oil and garlic. Buy a variety of herbs and spices. Experiment by adding the herbs to just a small portion of the vegetables in the pan. Sprinkling with sesame seeds adds to the visual appeal as well as the nutritional value.

Fruits – Use as a snack or as a side at breakfast. Make smoothies. Use real whipping cream and layer with fruit.

Whole Grains – Ezekiel bread, Near East wild rice or rice pilaf with almonds, stone ground whole wheat bread. Limit white starchy rice and potatoes while preparing to cleanse and dieting. They can over work the digestive tract. (Note: You get fiber from all of the above)

Meat and Dairy – Fish, chicken, turkey, and lamb. Use only lean beef. Variety is attained with the manner in which it is cut, the herbs or spices used, and the way it is presented on the plate.

Saturated Fat – Butter, meat, dairy, cheese, or coconut oil. Limit to 5 percent of your calories every meal.

Polyunsaturated Fat - You need equal amounts of omega 3 and omega 6.

> **Omega 3** - Omega 3 eggs, fish, fish oil, cod liver oil, canola oil, flaxseed oil, or ground flaxseed. Since Americans get too much omega 6, getting omega 3 is usually the area of greatest adjustment. We eat omega 3 eggs, eat fish for dinner once a week, and have tuna salad for lunch once a week. We also take fish oil every day. If you don't want to cook fish, go out for dinner and order salmon, walleye, tuna, or halibut.

> **Omega 6** – Raw nuts, seeds, legumes, grape seed oil, primrose oil, sesame oil, soybean oil, salad dressings, flax seed oil, and walnuts or walnut oil. I use olive oil for salad dressings and we eat raw nuts. Note: Nutritionists recommend taking cod liver oil, flax oil, and evening primrose oil every day.

Monounsaturated Fat – Olive oil, canola oil, almonds, avocados, and macadamia nuts. I lightly sauté with olive oil and make salad dressings with olive oil. Olives are a good snack if you think you have not gotten enough monounsaturated fat. Special note: Canola oil, and other vegetable oils can easily turn into Trans fats. I use olive oil (for cooking up to 325 degrees) because it's mentioned so often in scripture. I use coconut oil when cooking at higher temperatures.

Seeds and Nuts – Include in salads and vegetables. We like almonds and walnuts as a snack with fruit.

Herbs and Spices – Buy a different one every week and sprinkle it on just one portion of what's in your pan to see if you like it. Fresh or frozen herbs can be added at the last minute. I freeze fresh herbs, chop off what I need, and put the rest back in the freezer. I sprinkle a dried herb blend on my toast, and drizzle it with olive oil.

Sweets – For sugar, I use mainly honey. Try unrefined sugar (use sparingly). We also make fruit desserts.

Make yogurt and fruit smoothies. Try oatmeal cookies with raisins. Do not eat sweets while preparing to cleanse. Most nutritionists advise using Stevia or Xylo.

Liquids – Drink four 16 ounce glasses of water. Drink herbal teas (especially green tea) every day.

Drink one 6 to 8 ounce glass of fresh squeezed juice every morning.

ACHIEVING A BALANCED DIET

(Permission to print and tape this page inside your pantry along with the previous page)

The typical food pyramid can be arranged several different ways depending on which nutritionist you're talking to. However, most nutritionists, and nutrition minded doctors, agree that good carbs should be around 40 percent of your calories, protein should be around 30 percent of your calories, and good fats should make up the remaining 30 percent. How that translates into visual portion sizes on a plate can be difficult to figure out. I saw a diagram which was a great help. I've adapted it to agree with the books I read.

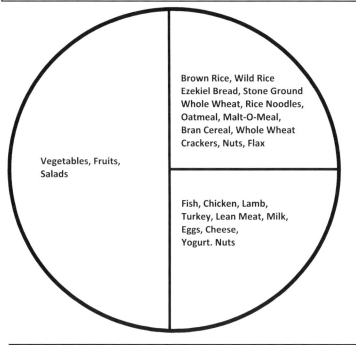

Vegetables, Fruits, Salads

Brown Rice, Wild Rice Ezekiel Bread, Stone Ground Whole Wheat, Rice Noodles, Oatmeal, Malt-O-Meal, Bran Cereal, Whole Wheat Crackers, Nuts, Flax

Fish, Chicken, Lamb, Turkey, Lean Meat, Milk, Eggs, Cheese, Yogurt. Nuts

Include herbs, spices, seeds, and oils.

Daily Servings (Food Pyramid)
Fruit (2-4)
1/2 C fresh , 1/4 C dried, 1/2 C juice
Vegetables (3-5)
(Most nutritionists recommend eating unlimited vegetables with at least 50% raw)
1/2 C raw or cooked, 1 C leafy greens, 1/2 C juice
Liver Friendly Starches and Grains (3)
1 slice bread, 1/2 bun, 4 crackers, 1 C dry cereal, 1/2 C cooked cereal, 1/2 C rice, 1/2 C semolina pasta. One handful of nuts. Some dietitians recommend cutting back on grains and getting more fiber from vegetables and nuts.
Meat (2-3)
2 to 3 oz. meat, 2 eggs, 4 TB peanut butter, 1/2 C nuts
Dairy (2-3)
8 oz milk or yogurt, 2 slices cheese, 1 C cottage cheese, 1 C healthy ice cream
Good Fats: Coconut oil, olive oil, fish, flax.

Adjust portions according to your caloric needs. Also, some foods will serve to meet the requirements for more than one group. If you want to keep close track without thinking about it, copy the chart in Appendix D (like the one below). For 30 days, check off what you eat during the day. By the end of 30 days, you'll have a good handle on what you should be eating. Remember to avoid refined sugar, white flour, and starchy foods.

☐ Fruit	☐ Vegetable	☐ Grains	☐ Meat	☐ Dairy	☐ Sat Fat	☐ Herbs
☐ Fruit	☐ Vegetable	☐ Grains	☐ Meat	☐ Dairy	☐ Omega 3	☐ Seeds
☐ Fruit	☐ Vegetable	☐ Grains	☐ Meat	☐ Dairy	☐ Omega 6	☐ Spices
☐ Fruit	☐ Vegetable				☐ Monoun-saturated	☐ Nuts
	☐ Vegetable					

Avoid (if not eliminate):

Processed foods White flour
Refined White Sugar Fast foods
Coffee
High starch foods

Decrease:

Red meat
Dairy
Saturated fats
Chocolate

Eliminate:

Hydrogenated oils / Trans fats
Anything God did not give to us as food
Deep fried foods
Preserved meats, lunchmeats
Processed vegetable oils
Colas, decaffeinated coffee
Aspartame
All Sugar (if you have arthritis or allergies)

Detoxification Organs in the Digestive Tract

Once you have achieved a healthy diet, it is time to think about detoxing (cleansing your digestive tract). God created our bodies with detoxification organs which eliminate toxins. These organs include the intestines, the liver, the kidneys, the lymphatic system, the lungs, and the skin. Following are detox organs which are part of our digestive system. Making sure they receive the nutrients God intended for them and keeping them free of pollutants are major keys to our health. Following is a very brief explanation of how each organ contributes to our overall health. (Colbert, 2003. 21-39)

1. **The Mouth** – In the mouth, saliva breaks food down with enzymes (some are manufactured by the body, some are in the food we eat). Chewing thoroughly ensures that food is broken down enough to prepare it for the stomach. Not chewing properly overworks the stomach. Chewing also causes white blood cells to be released which will attack harmful bacteria that may be in the food.

2. **The Stomach** – The stomach breaks food down with hydrochloric acid to prepare the food for the small intestines. Drinking more than 4 to 8 ounces of liquid with meals dilutes digestive juices so food is not broken down. Cold food and beverages decrease the activity of cells and slows down digestion.

3. **The Small Intestine** – Every tissue in our body is fed by our blood. The small intestines remove nutrients and pass them through the intestinal wall to be absorbed by blood vessels to transport them to organs. If our intestines are dirty, so are our blood and organs. Fiber passes on to the large intestine to remove waste.

4. **The Liver** – The liver has numerous functions. It is the key organ for metabolism and cleansing. It filters your blood and removes toxins from your body – if it is working properly. Nutrients are received by the liver, and sent to the rest of the body for absorption through the blood. Toxins are also filtered out in the liver, combined with bile, and sent back to the intestines to be excreted. In this way, the liver acts like a garbage man. If toxins aren't broken down by the liver they pile up like garbage. The liver metabolizes proteins and controls hormones. The lymphatic system is a secondary circulatory system under the skin (where cellulite forms). If the liver is over-worked, the lymphatic system will have difficulty ridding the body of fat and toxins (leaving you overweight and sluggish).

5. **The Large Intestines** – Fiber and water from the small intestine, combine with bile from the liver to remove waste. Not enough bile, fiber, or water can cause hard stools to remain in the body too long. If this happens, toxins can be reabsorbed back into the body (Colbert, 2003. 21-39).

Bacteria in the intestines: Most of the immune system is in the small intestine. Bad bacteria, good bacteria, and yeast exist like a balance of power (anarchy is bad). Overuse of antibiotics can kill both good and bad bacteria, so yeast grows out of control and can cause psoriasis, eczema, hives, diarrhea, bloating, and gas. Bad bacteria can become resistant to antibiotics and grow out of control creating poisons which damage cell membranes. They can even inactivate digestive enzymes. During cleansing, it is important to restore good bacteria to your intestines. The plan for doing so is included in the instructions for cleansing.

Another cleansing organ is the skin which excretes toxins through perspiration. I addition, the kidneys cleanse our body by continually discarding dead cells. But before going into detail about the actual process of cleansing, it's important to mention two other things I learned from the research I did. They are 1) the role enzymes play in digestion and health, and 2) the need for a balance of acid and alkaline in the stomach.

DIGESTION CAN BE HINDERED BY A LACK OF ENZYMES
Health is not just a matter of "You are what you eat."   It is, "You are what you digest."

What God created enzymes to do for us:	Food Sources:
Enzymes are found in all living cells. **Three types of enzymes are:** 1. Food 2. Digestive 3. Metabolic (rebuild the body) ♦ **Food Enzymes** are found in raw foods. Over cooking food destroys them. ♦ **Digestive Enzymes** are secreted by the body along the digestive tract to break down food. They take proteins, fats, and carbohydrates and restructure them so our body can use the nutrients in the food. ♦ **Metabolic Enzymes** speed up chemical reactions in the cells. They assist all bodily functions like stimulating the brain and repairing tissue. All of these work together for your health and vitality.	Making sure you eat a variety of fresh food and chewing your food thoroughly are crucial to the release of enzymes so food can be processed to nourish your body. ♦ Pineapple and papaya break up proteins. ♦ Avocados, bananas, mangos, alfalfa sprouts, barley grass, broccoli, and dark greens are high in enzymes. ♦ Beets aid digestion. ♦ Lactase enzyme supplements help digest milk. ♦ Overcooked starchy vegetables and pastas lack enzymes so they make the body work harder. ♦ Pancreatin is an enzyme supplement for food allergies. ♦ Eat 50% raw and 50% cooked vegetables for a balance of enzymes. Eggs have the enzyme, lecithin. ♦ Fresh squeezed juices have enzymes; however, the pasteurization of bottled juices destroys enzymes.

Health Notes: Cooking food at more than 118 degrees can kill almost all enzymes. When food enzymes are destroyed, the body must draw from metabolic (body building) enzymes to make more digestive enzymes. This can degenerate the body. However, cooking vegetables to a certain point makes them more readily digestible. Sprouting seeds and nuts helps increase the amount of enzymes that will be released. Simply soak them for one hour and then lay them flat to dry. For more information read *Prescription for Nutritional Healing* (2000. 59-62) or go to enzymedica.com.

DIGESTION CAN BE HINDERED BY AN ACID/ALKALI IMBALANCE

An imbalance of acid and alkaline can prevent your body from absorbing nutrients and can lead to disease. Health food stores usually have test strips for checking pH (Potential Hydrogen) levels. Signs of an imbalance are frequent sighing, water retention, migraine headaches, arthritis, dry hard stools, halitosis, and joint pain (Balch, 2000. 122-125). It may also lead to weight gain. Acids can also cause you to lose calcium. Citrus fruits which contain acids actually turn to alkaline in the body. A good rule to maintain a balance is to eat 80 percent alkaline-forming foods and 20 percent acid-forming foods. (See below)

Alkaline-Forming foods (80%)	DAIRY	Acid-Forming foods (20%)	NUTS
MOST FRESH FRUITS	Non Fat Milk	**FRUIT**	Cashews
Dates	**RAW NUTS**	Cranberries	Walnuts
Grapes	Almonds	Strawberries	Peanuts
Citrus	Brazil	**VEGETABLES**	Pecans
Apples	Nuts	Beans	Macadamia nuts
Bananas	**SEEDS**	**GRAINS**	**SEEDS**
Cherries	All sprouted seeds	Brown Rice	Pumpkin
Peaches	**BEANS**	Barley	Sesame
Pears	Soy	Wheat	Sunflower
Plums	Lima	Oats	Flax
Pineapples	Sprouted	Rye Breads	**BEANS**
Raspberries	**OILS**	**MEAT AND DAIRY**	Navy
Raisins	Olive	All Meats	Kidney
Melons	Soy	Milk	**FATS**
MOST VEGETABLES	Sesame	Cheese	Nuts
Too many to list	Corn	Eggs	Butter
GRAINS	**HONEY**	Fish	Cream
Buckwheat			All SUGARS
Corn			

CLEANSING YOUR BODY

(Consult your doctor before cleansing)

Before discussing cleansing, I want to define some terms I use so there will be no confusion:

♦ **Cleansing** – Ridding the body of toxic buildup.

♦ **Major Cleanse** – A cleanse that focuses on riding the body of toxins within a short period of time. Includes eating healthy and taking supplements specifically aimed at cleansing. It may, or may not, include juicing.

♦ **Juice Cleanse** – Going without food for a short period of time and drinking freshly squeezed juices for the purpose of resting the liver and cleansing. May be part of a major cleanse, a fast, or done two days every month as its own cleanse (recommended by most nutritionists).

♦ **Juicing** – Simply drinking fresh squeezed juices on a consistent basis for overall health.

♦ **Fasting** – Going without food in some manner for the purpose of seeking God. May or may not be part of a cleanse.

The first signs that something is wrong (indicating a need to cleanse) may include:

Hard stools only once a day. Stools should be soft but formed, and two to three times a day.

"Foggy-brain" and fatigue.

Body aches and joint pains.

Discoloring of skin or skin rashes.

Most of the doctors I read recommend that you do major cleanses no more than twice a year. Too many major cleanses can rid your body of good bacteria. However, in addition to doing two major cleanses, they do advise adding a juice fast once a month for two days (no additional supplements).

They also recommend that you refrain from using purge cleanses too often which can break toxins down too fast and they may not be excreted from your body. These toxins can be stored in your body, producing the opposite effect of what you're trying to do.

Caution: Some doctors recommend that you not fast if you have cancer, anemia, congestive heart failure, mental illness, kidney disease, liver disease, or you are pregnant or nursing. Talk to a nutrition- ally minded doctor about any cleanse or juicing.

Again, the purpose of this notebook is to help us eat right. It is not medical advice for treating specific disorders. However, there is a book (which I have talked about previously) that will help you. *Prescription for Nutritional Healing* includes extensive discussions about numerous disorders. It's a reference guide to drug-free remedies. Included in these remedies is advice as to what type of cleanse or fast can be done for individual disorders. This book is not "faith based," but it is an easy to understand, practical guide, from the perspective of a doctor and a nutritionist.

Before discussing the details of two major cleanses that I have learned about, and done for myself, I want to mention that some doctors recommend a more long term approach to cleansing. Simply go on the healthy eating program, drink fresh squeezed juices, and take a multivitamin that includes cleansing herbs. You may also want to take antioxidant supplements in addition to vitamins. Speak with a nutritionist or a doctor who is familiar with natural remedies.

Some doctors and nutritionists advise doing the following, no matter what major cleanse you choose:

♦ **Do a juice cleanse every month for one to three days.** Drink juices for these days (no additional supplements). Even if you do a major cleanse twice a year, and remain on a healthy diet, they believe once a month juice cleansing keeps your body clean and well supplied with nutrients. Com- bine it with a spiritual fast, and you'll benefit both physically and spiritually.

♦ **Drink fresh squeezed juices every morning of your life** (along with eating healthy and taking supplements) especially for chronically ill patients.

3 TYPES OF CLEANSES

The first cleanse we chose (recommended by Dr. Colbert's in *Toxic Relief* (2003. 43-58) advises:

1. Eat a healthy diet for two weeks to help rest your liver. While on this diet, do the following:
   - Drink a freshly squeezed vegetable or fruit juice drink every morning while eating a healthy diet. (Juicing separates nutrients from the pulp so they are easily digested and assimilated. Juice recipes are on page 83.)
   - Take supplements to support your liver while on this diet.
        Supplements recommended by Dr. Colbert while you are on your two week diet prior to cleaning include:
        a. Comprehensive multivitamin (take with meals)
        b. Comprehensive antioxidant
        c. Milk thistle (protects the liver from toxins)
        d. Amino Acid such as N-acetyl-cystein, "NAC" (raises the body's own level of glutathione)
        e. Lecithin (thins bile so the liver can detox easily, and also breaks down fat)
        f. Lactobacillus acidophilus (raises the level of good bacteria in your small intestine to aid your immune system)
        g. Fiber supplement (binds toxins and sweeps the colon clean) Make sure you drink plenty of water. It's important to avoid constipation so you may want an herbal laxative on hand.
        h. Green Superfood (a powdered drink mix which equals six servings of vegetables and herbs) We simply ate a good amount of 50 percent raw and 50 percent cooked vegetables and a salad every day. However, if I had a chronic illness, I would take Green Superfood. Check with your health food store or go to drcolbert.com.
   - Drink four 16 oz glasses of filtered water every day.
   - Get plenty of fiber.
2. At the end of two weeks, for one day, eat only fruits and vegetables.
3. The next day, begin a juice fast for two - three days (recipes on page 83). Take no supplements during this time. Drink a juiced drink 4 times each day. Continue to drink four - 16 oz. glasses of water.
4. The first day after your juice fast eat fresh fruit every two – three hours (no papaya or pineapple).
5. The second day after your juice fast eat the following:
        Breakfast – fruit
        Lunch and Dinner – fresh vegetable soup
6. The third day after your fast – in addition to soup, add a potato or salad with whole grain bread.
7. The fourth day after your fast – add chicken.
8. Eat a healthy diet for another two weeks. Reintroduce supplements until you run out and then take a multivitamin plus any others recommended by your doctor. We take a vitamin regiment recommended by our chiropractor (tailored to meet our health concerns). A health coach from our local health food store recommends taking: 1) a whole-foods based multivitamin with enzymes 2) fish oil such as cod liver oil 3) green super-food, and 4) liquid magnesium. From what I have studied, this seems to be an excellent recommendation.

After six months, I felt I needed another major cleanse and chose one recommended by Phyllis Balch in *Prescription for Nutritional Healing*: I took Ultimate Cleanse by Nature's Secret. This cleanse comes with a CD which is both educational and instructional. It has one bottle of cleansing herbs that release toxins from your body's tissues and organs. Another bottle contains fiber herbs that remove the toxins out of your body (I had to cut the fiber tablet in half). Ask your doctor, nutritionist, or health food store consultant if they can recommend a cleanse program for you to suit your state of health.

Special note: I learned first-hand that one thing most of these doctors said was absolutely true. You will likely feel tired during a major cleanse. Your conditions may even seem to worsen before they get better because toxins are being released from your system. Once your body has been rid of the "waste buildup," your body will have a better chance of healing itself.

In case you become constipated during your three days of cleansing, some nutritionists advise having an herbal laxative on hand. Some recommend that you use an enema. Remember, a backed up colon can release toxins back into your system, defeating your purpose. Vitamin C, drinking plenty of water, magnesium citrate powder, and taking a walk can also stimulate a bowel movement.

In addition to advice on cleansing, Dr. Colbert's book *Toxic Relief* contains a journal for spiritual fasting. In the same way that you can do a physical fast to cleanse your body, spiritual fasting can cleanse your spirit. Dr. Colbert has also written *What You Don't Know May Be Killing You*, and *The What Would Jesus Eat Cookbook*. Dr. Colbert also has a series of booklets for individual disorders called *The Bible Cure Books*. For more information go to www.drcolbert.com.

Jordan Rubin's books, *The Maker's Diet* and *Restoring Your Digestive Health*, detail a holistic approach which can be used by anyone who wants to see a dramatic change in their health within 40 days. If I had a chronic illness, I'd try everything he recommends in his book. He literally went from certain death to great health through the lifestyle changes he made. For more information go to www.golcommunications.com.

In addition to the above books, I would recommend that you read *The Bible Cure* by Dr. Cherry. The thing I learned the most from Dr. Cherry is to seek God for what Dr. Cherry calls, "your pathway to healing." Because everything can seem a little overwhelming, it's important to pray and ask God for His direction.

All of the doctors I read recommend doing a water-only fast only under the supervision of a physician. That's because water only fasting can release toxins from tissues so quickly that the body cannot excrete them efficiently. These toxins can end up back in the brain, spinal cord, and nerve tissues. That does not mean you should never do a water-only fast if you are sure it's the direction of the Lord. Even animals will fast near water when they are ill. However, they advise that you be under the care of your doctor at the time.

Remember, this isn't a cure-all. Every person deals with his or her own health concerns. Be an active participant in your health care and in deciding how many changes you need to make. Keep in mind there's healthy, healthier and healthiest. If you have a chronic disorder, you may want to make more drastic changes and obtain reading material which focuses on that ailment. The *Dummies* books (i.e. *Arthritis for Dummies*) are very informative. I know the name may be a little insulting, but I found them easy to understand (no jokes, please).

Finally, staying motivated can be difficult. It takes time, but remember, your body didn't become "clogged" overnight. And it will take time for your body to restore itself. The amazing truth is that God designed it to do just that – if we give our body the tools it needs to do so. Even then, we still deal with environmental toxins. But now, after just seven months of changing our habits, we're on the offensive. Anytime I'm tempted to return to old habits, I remind myself of what it felt like to have allergies and body aches.

JUICING

Because much of our food supply is depleted of nutrients, and because of the amount of toxins we are faced with daily, we need an abundance of healing nutrients from more vegetables and fruits than we would normally consume during a day. For instance, most of us would not eat a lemon, a bowl of berries and four oranges at one time. Juicing enables you to receive those needed nutrients. It also relieves your digestive tract from having to remove the pulp from the food.

To use juicing as part of a detox do the following: After being on a liver friendly diet for two weeks, make a list of the ingredients below according to the drinks you choose to use while detoxing. Run them through a juicer. The following recipes are sample Juice Drinks for Cleansing (from *Toxic Relief* by Dr. Colbert (2003. 87-89):

Breakfast

1 small lemon	4 carrots
1 bowl berries	1 handful of parsley
4 oranges, peeled	4 apples

Midmorning snack

2 carrots	1/2 cantaloupe
2 celery stalks	1 C berries
1 apple	
1 beet	

Lunch

Handful of parsley	2 stalks of celery
1 tomato	2 carrots
1 cucumber	1 beet
2 stalks of celery	1 handful broccoli 1/2 garlic clove

Evening – warm as a soup

4 carrots	1 cucumber
2 celery stalks	2 tomatoes
Handful of parsley	Parsley
1/2 clove of fresh garlic	1/2 clove of fresh garlic

In addition to including juicing as part of a major cleanse, it's a good idea to incorporate these into your normal eating routine. If you don't want to mess with juicing, you might want to try including a health shake of your choice (consult with your doctor or health food store).

Refreshing Drink for Cleansing and Boosting your Metabolism (from Dr. OZ)

Lemonade/ Limeade

Squeeze 2 lemons or limes (or a combination of both) into a glass. Sweeten with Truvia sweetener or Stevia

Add ice

You can also include a few dashes of hot sauce which will increase your metabolism – and add a little kick. At this point you can fill the glass with filtered water or seltzer water for a fizz.

HANDY FOOD CHART
(It may be helpful to take this to the grocery store with you, along with your shopping list.)

Food Guide	Limit	Include
Beans	Canned	Fresh or frozen (all cooked without pork fat)
Beverages	Coffee, cocoa, sweetened juices, soda pop, black tea	Filtered water, herbal tea, fresh vegetable and fruit juices
Dairy Products	Soft cheeses, artificially colored, pasteurized cow's milk	Goat cheese, low fat cottage cheese, natural yogurt, goat's milk (most like "mother's milk") buttermilk
Eggs	Fried	Omega 3 (boiled, poached or sautéed in olive oil)
Fish	Fried, shellfish, salted, anchovies, herring, canned in oil	Freshwater white fish such walleye and halibut, salmon (broiled, baked or sautéed in olive oil) water-packed tuna
Fruits	Canned, bottled with sweeteners	Fresh, frozen, stewed, or dried without sweeteners
Grains	White flour, white rice, pasta, crackers, instant oatmeal.	Whole grains: cereals, breads, muffins, crackers, cream of wheat or rye cereal, buckwheat, millet, oats, brown rice, wild rice (Kashi brand crackers and La Tortilla wraps are free of trans fats)
Meats	Limit beef hot dogs, lunchmeat, corned beef, duck, spare ribs, gravies	Turkey, chicken, lamb, wild game, lean beef
Nuts	Salted or roasted, peanuts (if allergic)	Handful of fresh raw almonds, macadamia, pistachios, walnuts
Oils	Limit saturated fats. No hydrogenated oils, no shortening, no margarine	Cold-pressed olive, coconut, safflower, sesame, flaxseed, and sunflower oils
Seasonings	Black or white pepper, table salt	Garlic, onions, spices, herbs, dried vegetables, vinegar, tamari, sea salt (contains vitamins and minerals), kosher salt
Soups	Canned, fat stock, creamed	Homemade bean, lentil, pea, vegetable, barley, brown rice, onion, chicken, beef, stocks
Sprouts, seeds	Any cooked in high heat	All raw, sprouted, lightly toasted
Sweets	White, brown, or raw sugar, corn syrups, chocolate, candy, syrups, jams, jellies, Splenda	Barley malt or rice syrup, raw honey, pure maple syrup, unsulfured blackstrap molasses, Stevia
Vegetables and Greens	Any with added salt or preservatives. Iceberg Lettuce	All raw, fresh, frozen (no additives). Do not overcook. Use romaine, spinach, and dark leafy greens. (They are more nutritious and higher in fiber.)

Shopping Tips:

♦ I write out my menu (keeping in mind our family history and health concerns). Then I make a grocery list from that menu. I keep the menu handy along with any recipes needed for the week.

♦ I shop around the outside edge of the grocery store first so we will be eating everything as fresh as possible. I try to buy items on the inside only with scrutiny. At first, I read nearly every label, but now I'm getting more of it memorized. If possible, I get things like mayo at the health food store. I also buy organic as much as my budget will allow. I rinse all thin skinned fruits and vegetables.

♦ Before purchasing an item, I stop and think about what it will do the cells inside my body (and those of my family).

Note: Frozen is sometimes better than fresh, depending on the season. Fresh vegetables are often picked green, but frozen are picked ripe and frozen right away. Frozen are also cut for you, saving time. Jordan Rubin has a video on how to shop healthy (golcommunications.com).

Notes (write down your plan for detoxing)

6 - COOKING HEALTHY MADE EASY

I've had people ask me for a menu (along with the recipes) that would teach them how to balance out what I have learned about cooking healthy. So I did my best to think through all the requirements and came up with a menu which you will find in this chapter. The recipes for the menu are for two people. I have kept them fairly simple on purpose. Make adjustments according to your taste. I have also included a few extra recipes, just in case you may not like something on the menu. There is also a page with an alternative menu which does not require recipes.

You'll notice that the recipes do not have page numbers. This allows you to add your own recipes to this book. You may want to purchase dividers for easy reference. I began by adapting recipes I had used previously. Then, I set a goal of making one new dish every week. For more recipes you may want to purchase a copy of The What *Would Jesus Eat Cook Book* by Don Colbert, M.D., *Nourishing Traditions* by Sally Fallon, or *The Lazy Person's Whole Food Cookbook* by Stephen Byrnes.

Helpful Hints:
◆ Refer to your "My Plan" Sheet for any changes you have chosen to make in your eating habits.
◆ Purchase any supplements you may need for doing the cleanse you chose.
◆ After reading this chapter, decide which menu you want to use for cooking healthy. A grocery list has been provided for you in Appendix B.
◆ Keep the menu and the recipes for the week in this notebook. Keep them handy and you won't have to think about what you're going to make that day.
◆ Shop around the outside edge of the grocery store first, where everything is fresh or frozen. Read labels carefully for those items purchased from inside aisles. Those are the items you may want to purchase from a health food store.
◆ Two weeks before your cleanse begin eating healthy. (The three days you choose for doing a cleanse should be a time when you can get some rest.)

Cooking Tips:
∗ Nutrients in food can be depleted by exposure to high heat, light, air and water. It is best to steam or lightly sauté vegetables. Reserve any liquid as it will contain some of the water soluble nutrients. Pour the liquid over what was cooked or use it as a broth. It is also helpful to use a lid as much as possible. Cut everything in as big of sizes as possible, taking the recipe into account.
∗ Chop everything right before beginning to cook. Pre-measure spices and herbs and put the ingredients in small dishes. When it comes time to cook, you can just toss them in. It's much easier.
∗ I very rarely measure. Get creative – cooking is not a strict science.

Cooking with Children:
Have your children help you measure spices and herbs. You do the chopping. Then, when it comes time to cook, they can help you add the ingredients. They will learn to measure and cook at the same time. Children can also tear the lettuce for the salad. Have them count out the nuts and fruit slices. It's not that you need a certain number of nuts or fruits, but it will give them something to do and help with their math skills.

Remember the three rules to ask yourself when shopping:
1. Is this included in what God gave us for food?
2. Has it been chemically altered by man?
3. Am I making this food my god?

(I highly recommend reading Dr. Russell's book, *What the Bible Says About Healthy Living*.)

And whatever you do, do not get stressed out. It takes time, so be patient with yourself. Making these changes gradually kept us encouraged to continue with our goal to go from healthier toward healthiest. You may want to simple adapt your own recipes to the health guides mentioned previously.

MENU FOR ONE WEEK (A shopping list for this menu is in Appendix B)

This menu includes all four food groups, nuts, seeds, herbs and spices for seven days. If you're concerned about cholesterol, be sure to cook eggs with coconut oil and garlic (both reduce bad cholesterol). You can also substitute yogurt and fruit for eggs one day. If you're using this as a liver friendly diet in preparing to cleanse, you should include a juiced drink every morning before your water. **Don't forget to drink four – 16 ounce glasses of water. If you forget a glass in between meals, when you begin to cook, drink it then (don't forget your family).**

DAY ONE

Breakfast – Eggs with Vegetables, Carrot/Orange Slices, Toast (I also love spinach with my eggs)

Lunch – Turkey Burgers served open faced, Basic Lettuce Salad

Dinner – Lemon Pepper Chicken, Broccoli/Carrots, Near East Rice Pilaf

Snack – Apple with a handful of Almonds and/or Walnuts.

DAY TWO

Breakfast – Cinnamon Oatmeal, Fresh Fruit (I eat a TB of natural peanut butter as a protein with my carb)

Lunch – Basic Salad (with chicken chunks from day one), Fresh Carrots, Wheat Crackers

Dinner – Basic Fish Recipe, Green Beans with Red Peppers, Parsley Potatoes

Snack – Banana Raspberry Smoothie, Handful of Nuts

DAY THREE

Breakfast – Omega 3 Eggs Boiled with Chives, Toast, Fresh Fruit, Carrot or Spinach

Lunch – Fat Burning Soup, Wheat Crackers

Dinner – Steak Smothered in Onions, Vegetable Medley, Mandarin Orange Salad, Rice

Snack – Orange with nuts

DAY FOUR

Breakfast – Cinnamon Oatmeal, Fresh Fruit, Alternative – Healthy Cereal

Lunch – Steak wrap with meat from previous day, Carrots

Dinner – Marinated Turkey Tenderloins, Bundle of Vegetables, Greek Salad, Rice

Snack – Cottage Cheese, Fresh Fruit and Nuts

DAY FIVE

Breakfast – Eggs with Seasoned Tomatoes or Eggs with Salsa, Toast, Fresh Fruit

Lunch – Vegetable Soup, Fresh Vegetables on the side, Whole Grain Crackers

Dinner – Italian Chicken Smothered in Tomatoes, Grilled Zucchini, Wild Rice

Snack – Berries in Yogurt, Nuts

DAY SIX

Breakfast – Cinnamon Oatmeal, Fresh Fruit

Lunch – Tuna Salad Wrap, Sweet Pepper Salad

Dinner – Tropical Island Chicken, Skewered Vegetables, New Potatoes

Snack – Celery with Natural Peanut Butter, Crackers

DAY SEVEN

Breakfast – Healthy cereal, Toast, Fresh Fruit

Lunch – Soup (whatever is left from the previous days), Fresh Vegetables, Crackers

Dinner – Turkey Meatloaf, Snap Peas with Carrots, Cucumber and Tomato Salad

Snack – Trail Mix

If dieting try eating the fat burning soup recipe every day for lunch. Limit starchy foods. Take lecithin. Use mustard and cayenne to raise metabolism. Read The Fat Flush by Ann Louise Gittleman MS, CNS (adapt this diet to agree with the three rules by Dr. Russell).

ALTERNATIVE EASY MENU
(Forget recipes - but stick with the healthy eating guidelines)

Keep the following herb and spice seasonings near the stove:

- Sea salt, pepper (both in a grinder)
- All purpose seasoning for vegetables, eggs, and meat; Mix together equal parts dried parsley, basil, oregano, lemon pepper, celery salt, and paprika. Purchase them at your health food store – it's less expensive.
- Italian Seasoning

(McCormick makes their own All Purpose Seasoning and Italian Seasoning which are also very tasty.)

Sample Seasonings to use on Meat:

Prepared seasonings such as Mexican, Asian, and Cajun mixes

Use your favorite prepared blend. Just read the label to make sure it does not have extra salt, preservatives, or hydrogenated oils.

Breakfast

Eggs, oatmeal, cereal with fruit, yogurt with fruit and toast, or just fruit and toast.

- Season eggs with one herb at a time to try it out. Always include a fresh vegetable. Boil, sauté, or scramble the eggs for variety. Try dill (or another herb) on boiled eggs. Sauté some tomatoes, garlic and onion in olive oil. Sprinkle with herbs. Either pour eggs over the cooked vegetables and scramble, spoon tomatoes over the cooked eggs, or have the tomatoes on the side. Include green pepper and mushrooms for variety.
- Cinnamon Oatmeal (see recipe)
- Toast sprinkled with all purpose seasoning and drizzled with olive oil, or drizzle with honey.

Lunch

- Make two soups on the weekend or buy soup at the health food store (recipes included).
- Make a salad or tortilla wrap sandwich using the meat from the previous day's dinner. Heat meat, shred it for sandwiches, and throw in some sweet peppers, and onions.
- Have fresh vegetables or fruit on the side.
- Eat crackers with soup if not having a sandwich (Kashi brand crackers and Triscuits do not contain hydrogenated oils.)

Dinner

- **Vegetable** – Keep a variety of frozen vegetables on hand. Buy both individual and combination vegetables. Simply steam or sauté in olive oil and garlic. If sautéing, add an herb.
- **Meat** – Season with one of the above seasonings. Find variety by the way it's sliced. Skewer along with vegetables for the grill. Plate creatively. Put meat on rice. If you have not had a salad for lunch, have it at dinner. Make extra meat to have for lunch the next day. Puree some vegetables to use as a sauce for meats.
- **Wild rice or potato (limit potatoes)** – Buy varieties of Near East rice. For variety serve whole wheat bread in place of rice.

Snack – Use your snack to make up for anything you did not have during the day.

- Fruit, fresh vegetables, yogurt and fruit, cottage cheese and fruit, or nuts.

Helpful Hint: I thaw frozen berries in a container and keep them in the refrigerator. I drain a spoonful and scoop them into some yogurt nearly every day for lunch or a snack. Sometimes, I sweeten the juice slightly and drink it.

BEEF RECIPES

(Eat red meat only once a week – if at all – while preparing for a major cleanse.)

Pepper Steaks

1/2 – 3/4 LB round steak, cut in strips

2 T coconut oil

1 1/4 C beef stock

1 t stevia or raw sugar

1 t curry powder

1/2 t salt

1 green pepper sliced

1 medium onion cubed

1 - 2 T cornstarch mixed with 2 T water

1 tomato chopped

Brown meat. Add stock, water, sweetener, curry powder and salt. Boil and simmer 1 hour. Add vegetables. Stir in cornstarch mixture. Add tomatoes. Serve over brown rice.

Roast

3 LB lean roast

1 medium onion sliced

Salt and pepper

Cook in crock pot according to directions. Keep roast in the freezer, along with frozen mixed veggies to make a quick vegetable beef soup. Use leftovers for sandwiches.

Steak Smothered in Onions (limit to a small quantity)

2 lean steaks seasoned with pepper and salt

 Coconut oil

1 garlic clove

½ Onion sliced

Rub steak with oil and garlic clove. Season with pepper and salt. Sauté in olive oil. Remove when done. Add sliced onions to the pan along with a pat of real butter. Cook onions until brown in color and serve on top of the steak.

Puree and drizzle over grilled meat:

For beef puree: mushrooms, shallots, and beef stock

For chicken puree: spinach, garlic, and herbs

For fish: tomatoes and basil (Add any herb blend of your choice)

BREAKFAST RECIPES

(If watching cholesterol, combine one whole egg with just the yolk of another egg.)

Cinnamon Oatmeal

1 C milk

1 C of old fashioned oatmeal (preferably from a health food store)

1/4 t cinnamon

2 T ground flaxseeds

1 T honey or raw sugar for sweetener Frozen or fresh blueberries (optional)

Grind flaxseeds in a coffee grinder (Don't use pre-ground). Pour milk into saucepan. Add oatmeal. Cook until thick and bubbly. Lower heat. Cook about 5 more minutes until thick. Add flaxseeds, sweetener, and berries. Be sure to drink water or the flaxseeds will bind you.

Eggs, Boiled with Chives

1 boiled omega 3 egg

Top with chopped chives and drizzle with olive oil

Eggs with Salsa

3 – 4 omega 3 eggs

1 T olive oil

Scramble eggs lightly

Top with salsa

Eggs with Seasoned Tomatoes

3 – 4 omega 3 eggs

All-purpose dried herbs, or your own favorite blend of herbs

8 – 10 cherry tomatoes halved

1 small garlic clove

Olive oil

Whip eggs. Drizzle olive oil in a non-stick pan. Sauté garlic. Pour eggs into pan. Fold over to one side of the pan. Sauté tomatoes on the other side of pan. Sprinkle both with herbs. Season with salt and pepper. Scoop eggs onto a plate and top with tomatoes.

Simply Organic (found at most health food stores) has an all-purpose seasoning that is delicious and can be used in just about any egg, vegetable, or chicken dish.

Eggs with Veggies (If you have "picky eaters," try adding just one new veggie or herb every time you make eggs and do a "taste" test.)

3 whole omega 3 eggs, plus 1 egg white

1 small green onion chopped

3 – 4 cherry tomatoes, or 1/4 C of Roma tomatoes

1/4 sweet red pepper chopped

2 – 3 shitake mushrooms chopped

1 small garlic clove chopped

Salt and pepper to taste

Basil, Italian seasoning, or All Purpose Herb Seasoning

1 T olive oil

Beat eggs in a bowl. Chop veggies and garlic. Heat a nonstick pan. Drizzle with olive oil.

Drop in veggies and sauté about two minutes. Pour eggs over veggies. Lift edges of eggs to let liquid go underneath. Season with salt and pepper. Turn. When almost done, sprinkle with herb of your choice. Sprinkle with shredded cheese if desired. Remove from heat. Put a lid over the eggs until cheese melts. (We use cheese sparingly)

Flax Buttermilk Pancakes

1 C whole wheat flour

1/4 C flax seed meal

1/2 t soda

2 t baking powder

1/2 t salt

1 T honey

1 omega 3 egg

1 C buttermilk

1 T coconut or olive oil

Combine dry ingredients. Mix egg, milk, and oil. Add dry ingredients. Spray a griddle and cook pancakes. Top with strawberries, hot cinnamon applesauce, or peaches sweetened with honey.

Toast

Sprinkle dried herb blend on toast while hot and drizzle with olive oil

Alternative Breakfast:

Yogurt with fruit (thaw frozen fruit and scoop drained fruit into yogurt.) Serve with toast.

DESSERT RECIPES

(Only the Melon Shake and the Yogurt Dessert are allowed while preparing for a cleanse)

Chocolate Chip (or Raisin) Oatmeal, Nut Cookies

1 C butter (or 1/2 C butter and 1/2 C coconut oil)

3/4 C honey

1 omega 3 eggs

1/4 C natural almond butter or natural peanut butter

1 t vanilla

Cream above together then add

2 C whole wheat flour, for a smoother texture use half unbleached flour 2 C oatmeal

1 t soda

1/2 t salt

1 – 1 1/2 C raisins (or chocolate chips)

1 C chopped nuts

Combine ingredients. Drop on cookie sheet. Bake at 350 about 8 minutes.

Melon Shake

1 C watermelon cubed

1 C cantaloupe cubed

1 C honeydew melon cubed

1 C yogurt

2 T lemon juice

1/2 t vanilla extract

1/2 C crushed ice

Combine melons and process in a smoothie machine or blender. Blend in yogurt, lemon juice, vanilla, and crushed ice. Process until smooth.

(See page 188 of *The What Would Jesus Eat Cookbook* by Don Colbert)

Yogurt with Fruit

Thaw frozen berries, drain and reserve liquid. Layer alternately in a sundae dish with yogurt. Drizzle berry juice over the dessert.

FISH RECIPES

Basic Fish Recipe

2 fish fillets

Fresh squeezed lemon juice

Salt and pepper

Paprika or lemon pepper (optional)

Coconut oil

If fish smells a little fishy, soak in milk one hour. Drain and pat dry. Drizzle with lemon juice. Season. Sauté in coconut oil.

Parsley and Dill Snapper

1 LB snapper seasoned with salt and pepper

1/2 C vegetable broth (may use chicken stock)

2 T parsley

1 T green onion chopped

1 T fresh dill

1/4 C fresh lemon juice plus lemon zest (grated skin of a lemon)

Mix ingredients, except lemon juice. Pour over snapper. Drizzle with lemon juice. Roast 15-25 minutes at 300 degrees.

Salmon Patties

1 small can salmon

1 omega 3 egg

1/4 C wheat crackers (crushed into crumbs)

1 green onion chopped

Drain salmon. Mix all ingredients. Make into patties. Season with salt and pepper. Sauté in coconut oil.

Fish with Mango Salsa

2 fish fillets seasoned with salt and pepper

1 C fresh mango chopped

2 T lime juice

1/4 C plum tomatoes chopped

1/4 C chopped red onion

1 T jalapeno pepper chopped and 1/4 C yellow pepper chopped

 1 T fresh cilantro chopped

Prepare fish according to basic fish recipe. Mix all remaining ingredients. Vary according to your own taste. Serve over fish.

POTATO AND RICE RECIPES

(If preparing for a major cleanse, go light on starchy foods – no white rice or potatoes.)

Brown Rice from Scratch

1 T olive oil

1 green onion chopped

1/2 C carrot chopped

1 C brown rice

2 1/2 – 3 C chicken stock (add more as needed)

1/2 t dried or 1 T fresh parsley, salt and pepper to taste

Sauté onions and carrots. Add rice. Cook 1 minute. Add chicken stock and bring to a boil. Reduce heat and simmer until stock is absorbed (about 1 hour). Add more stock as needed. Add parsley when tender and let stand 5 minutes.

Near East Rice - You can buy this at your health food store or Wal-Mart. It's all natural. It comes in handy for those who do not want to make rice from scratch. It has herbs so it is healthy. Make according to the directions using olive oil.

For more nutrition add chopped carrots, peas, chopped onion, or chopped mushrooms.

New potatoes

6 new potatoes, halved

2 T butter

1 T fresh parsley or 1 t dried

Fresh ground pepper Salt

Boil potatoes in salt water. When tender, drain. Add butter and parsley. Season with salt and pepper.

Wild Rice (Near East makes a wild rice)

2 1/2 – 3 C beef stock

1 C wild rice

Boil stock. Add rice. Reduce heat and simmer until stock is absorbed. Add more stock as needed.

POULTRY RECIPES

Chicken Fajitas

1 T olive oil

2 T lemon juice

1 1/2 t each of salt, dried oregano, and cumin

1 small garlic clove chopped

1/2 t paprika

1/2 t crushed red pepper flakes

4 boneless, skinless chicken breasts cut into strips

Mix first 6 ingredients. Pour into plastic bag. Add chicken and refrigerate overnight. Grill the next day. Sauté 1 green pepper, 1 red pepper, and 1 small onion. Add to grilled meat.

Italian Chicken Smothered in Tomatoes

(Don't forget to buy a whole chicken – cut up) and reserve the remainder for making salads, soups, or sandwiches)

2 chicken breasts with bones – seasoned with salt and pepper

2 T coconut oil

1 clove of garlic

1/2 small onion chopped

1/2 C green pepper chopped

1-2 tomatoes chopped Italian Seasoning

Drizzle olive oil in a pan. Sauté chicken until golden and brown. Remove from pan. Add a little more olive oil. Sauté garlic, onion, green pepper, and tomatoes. Sprinkle with Italian Seasoning. Cook for about 5 minutes (until slightly tender). Return chicken to the pan.

Lemon Pepper Chicken

Two chicken breasts on the bone seasoned with lemon pepper, salt and pepper

Coconut oil

1 garlic clove chopped

Season chicken with lemon pepper, salt and pepper. Grill or sauté in coconut oil with garlic.

Marinated Turkey Tenderloins

1/4 C soy sauce

1/4 C olive oil

1/4 C cooking sherry

2 T lemon juice

2 T crushed onion

1/4 t ground ginger

1 LB Turkey Breasts (boneless and skinless)

Mix first 6 ingredients. Marinate turkey for one hour. Grill.

Smothered Chicken Provolone

4 chicken breasts

2 T coconut oil

2 garlic cloves

Fresh ground pepper

1/2 C onion chopped

1/2 C shitake mushrooms chopped

1/2 C chicken stock

1 – 2 t cornstarch

1/2 C cooking wine (optional)

4 slices of provolone cheese

Sauté chicken in olive oil until done. Remove from pan and put in baking dish. Add more olive oil to pan. Sauté garlic, onion, and mushrooms until tender. Add chicken stock and cooking wine. Cook 5 minutes. Thicken with cornstarch. Pour over chicken. Cover chicken with cheese and bake at 350 until cheese is melted. If cleansing, omit cheese.

Tropical Island Chicken (It makes life easy when you marinate something the previous day.)

1/2 C soy sauce

1/3 C olive oil

1/4 C water

2 T dried minced onion

2 T sesame seeds

1 T raw sugar

3 garlic cloves minced

1/8 t ground ginger

1/2 t salt

Pinch of cayenne

4 chicken breasts (bone-in or boneless)

Combine all ingredients except chicken. Stir. Put chicken in a bag. Pour marinade over chicken. Refrigerate overnight. Drain. Grill.

Turkey Meatloaf

1 LB ground turkey

1 omega 3 egg

1 C tomato juice

3/4 C oats

1/4 C onion chopped

1/2 t salt

1/4 t ground pepper.

Combine all of the ingredients. Bake 40 min at 350 degrees. Drain excess fat. Top with BBQ sauce (read label for sugar content). Go light on the sauce in cleansing. Bake 20 more minutes.

Hint: When making salad dressing, combine all the ingredients except the oil. Whisk oil in slowly at the end to emulsify. Make additional to use all week.

Basic Lettuce Salad

Use a variety of leafy greens (refrain from using Ice berg lettuce as it's lower in nutrients)

Add whatever fresh veggies or fruit your family likes

Include seeds, nuts, parsley and alfalfa to taste

Basic Vinaigrette Dressing (Test by dipping a piece of lettuce into the dressing)

1/2 C red wine vinegar (Or one of your favorite vinegars)

One third as much oil (A little less than 1/4 of a cup)

Italian Seasoning or All Purpose Seasoning

1 garlic clove, chopped Salt and pepper

Cucumber and Tomato Salad

1 1/2 C cucumbers, thin sliced

1 1/2 C tomatoes chopped

1/2 C onions diced

1/2 C red wine vinegar

1 t dried dill weed

1 T raw sugar

Mix cucumbers, tomatoes, and onions. Mix remaining ingredients and pour over vegetables. Marinate one hour. Overnight is better.

Mandarin Orange Salad

2 T raw sugar

2 T cider vinegar

1 1/2 T orange juice concentrate (scoop from container and freeze the rest)

1 1/2 t. red wine vinegar

1 1/2 t chopped green onion

2 – 3 T olive oil

Combine all of the above and serve over romaine lettuce topped with one small can of mandarin oranges, sunflower seeds, and slivered almonds. You can also add chicken. (Frozen juice concentrates are not the healthiest for drinking, but in this small amount it's not a great concern.)

Strawberry, Avocado, and Walnut Salad

Spring Mix Lettuce

2 strawberries cut in quarters (also good with blueberries)

1/2 avocado cut into small squares

1/4 C walnut pieces

(Greek salad dressing from next page)

Greek Salad with Dill and Cilantro Salad Dressing

2 T red wine vinegar

2 T raw sugar

2 T parmesan cheese

1 small garlic clove, chopped

1/2 t dill (scant)

1/2 t cilantro (scant)

1 t Dijon mustard

Italian Seasoning to taste Salt and pepper

3 T olive oil

This is good served over a combination of cherry tomatoes, cucumber, yellow pepper, red onions, black olives, and feta or goat cheese.

Romaine, Walnut, and Goat Cheese Salad

Romaine lettuce and fresh spinach Walnuts

Goat or Feta cheese

Combine and use the dill and cilantro salad dressing from above

Sweet Pepper Salad

Romaine lettuce and fresh spinach (optional)

1/2 red, yellow and orange sweet peppers, chopped Sesame seeds

Use the mandarin orange salad dressing, a healthy vinaigrette, or dressing of your choice.

SANDWICH RECIPES

Basic Chicken Sandwich

Whole wheat bread

Shredded chicken Lettuce

Tomato

Fresh sweet red peppers

Mayo from health food store

Pita Sandwich

Make a sandwich using any of the meat from a previous meal

Examples: Tropical Island Chicken Pita, Roasted Red Pepper Chicken Pita, Add any veggies you like.

Sandwich Wraps (Use La Tortilla wraps – they have no Trans fats.)

Make a wrap using any meat from a previous dinner.

Include vegetables.

Examples – fajita wrap or chicken salad wrap.

Salmon Burgers – Open Faced

1 small can salmon

1 omega 3 egg

1/4 C whole wheat cracker crumbs

1 green onion chopped

Whole wheat buns

Drain salmon. Mix all ingredients. Make into patties. Season with salt and pepper. Sauté. Serve with dill sauce: 4 T butter, 1 green onion chopped, 1/2 t lemon zest, 2 T fresh squeezed lemon juice, 1/4 C chopped fresh dill, 1/4 t salt, freshly ground pepper. Serve on an open faced bun. Drizzle with dill sauce.

Tuna Salad Wrap

Make your favorite tuna salad

Serve in a whole wheat La Tortilla wrap

Turkey Burgers

1/2 LB ground turkey

1 slice onion chopped

1/2 carrot chopped (optional)

Salt and pepper to taste

Mix all ingredients. Serve on open faced whole wheat bun topped with tomato.

SNACK IDEAS

(Keep fresh fruit, nuts, or trail mix on the counter every day for snacking)

Apple or other fresh fruit with a handful of nuts.

Banana Raspberry Smoothie

1 sliced banana

1 1/4 C frozen raspberries

1/2 C low fat milk

Place banana in freezer for 10 minutes. Process banana and remaining ingredients in a blender until smooth.

Berries in Yogurt

1/4 C frozen berries

1 container of natural yogurt

Thaw and drain berries. Reserve liquid. Stir berries into yogurt. Drizzle liquid over yogurt mix. This makes a great dessert when layered in a small, clear sundae dish.

Eat with a handful of nuts.

Celery sticks with Natural Peanut Butter and Raisins.

Spread natural peanut butter on celery sticks and top with raisins

Cottage cheese topped with fresh peaches

Walnuts (either chop and put on top of peaches or eat separately)

Trail Mix

Purchase at your health food store.

Dried Berries

Purchase an assortment (They're also good in salads)

SOUP RECIPES

Anti-Cancer Soup (This recipe was given to me by a friend)
2 C hot water
1 green onions, chopped
2 T caraway seeds
2 carrots, chopped
2 slices (each) purple and green cabbage
2 C broccoli, chopped
1 red pepper, chopped
3 T dill weed
Soak caraway seeds in water (24 hours). Drain. Boil onions in 2 cups of water. Add remaining vegetables. Sprinkle with an all-purpose herb blend. Cook 5 minutes. Garnish with dill (or add to water).

Fat Burning Soup
6 large green onions, chopped
2 green peppers, chopped
1 or 2 large cans diced tomatoes
1 bunch celery, chopped
1 large head of cabbage, chopped
Italian seasoning
1 bay leaf
Salt and pepper to taste
1 pkg. Lipton dry onion soup mix
Mix all ingredients. Add enough water to cover. Cook until vegetables are tender.

Turkey or Chicken Noodle Soup (Vary to your own liking)
1 quart chicken stock (may need to add some chicken bouillon for flavor)
1/4 C onion, chopped
1 – 2 carrots, chopped
1/2 C frozen peas
3 shitake mushrooms, chopped
(You may use frozen vegetable mix in place of chopped vegetables for convenience)
Cubed leftover turkey or chicken from a previous day's supper
1/4 to 1/2 bag of whole grain noodles, or rice noodles
Pour stock into a sauce pan. Season with bouillon. Bring to a boil. Add vegetables. Season with all purpose seasoning. Add a bay leaf for more flavor. Simmer until veggies are almost done. Add noodles and continue to cook until done.

Vegetable Beef Soup (Vary according to your own liking)
1 small onion, chopped
2/3 LB roast, chunked (from a previous meal)
2 cans beef consommé (Use juice from cooking roast the previous day if you have it left).
2 small tomatoes, diced
2 carrots, chopped
1 potato, chopped
1 C frozen green beans
(In place of all the vegetables you can use a frozen mixed vegetable combination for convenience.)
1/4 t each dried thyme and chili powder

Broccoli with Carrots

1 small head of broccoli

2 carrots sliced into bite sized pieces Steam until just tender (do not overcook)

(For ease, buy a frozen carrot and broccoli mix and steam them)

Bundle of Veggies

1 T olive oil or coconut oil

1 T butter

1 garlic clove, chopped

1 green onion, chopped

Italian Seasoning

8 oz. shitake mushrooms, sliced

1 tomato, chopped (large chunks)

1 C sliced zucchini

1/2 t salt

Place ingredients on parchment paper (in the aisle with waxed paper). Season. Fold paper over beginning at one end and keep folding until you come to the other side. Seal with a paper clip. Bake about 20 – 25 minutes at 350 degrees.

Green Beans with Red Peppers

1 LB fresh green beans

1 red pepper, sliced

1 clove of garlic, chopped

Sliced almonds or sesame seeds

1 T olive oil (may need additional)

Salt and pepper

Blanch green beans (boil in water about 5 minutes). Drain. Sauté red peppers and garlic in olive oil. Add green beans. Season. Top with almonds and/or sesame seeds.

Grilled Zucchini

2 zucchini, sliced

1/4 to 1/2 inch thick lengthwise

Olive oil

1 tomato, chopped

1/4 onion, chopped

2 slices green pepper, chopped

1 garlic clove

Italian Seasoning Salt and pepper

Slice zucchini and vegetables. Chop garlic. Brush zucchini with olive oil and season with salt and pepper. Sauté in a pan or grill. Remove zucchini. Sauté remaining vegetables with garlic. Sprinkle with Italian seasoning. Serve sautéed vegetables over zucchini.

Skewered Vegetables with Herbs

Cherry Tomatoes Zucchini

Red onion

Red and green bell peppers Olive oil

Garlic salt

All purpose herb blend

Kosher salt

Cut vegetable in one inch chunks or slices. Alternate veggies on skewers. Brush with olive oil. Season and grill.

Snap Peas with Carrots

Snap pea and carrot mix from frozen food section Steam or sauté in olive oil and garlic.

Sweet Carrots

1 LB carrots sliced

3 T butter and/or olive oil

1 T honey or raw sugar

1 t Kosher salt

Place carrots in a pan with 1/2 inch water and remaining ingredients. Bring to a boil, reduce heat and simmer until done. Taste and adjust seasoning.

Vegetable Medley

1 yellow zucchini cut to bite size

1 sweet red pepper chopped

1 C sugar snap peas

2 T olive oil

1 medium garlic clove

Italian seasoning or lemon pepper

Cut vegetables any way you like. Sauté in olive oil. Add garlic and Italian seasoning. Sprinkle with sesame seeds.

Notes (summarize your commitment for change)

APPENDIX A

Dr. Russell's "other principle" (continued from pages 5-11)

One of the biggest questions I get asked when teaching a seminar is, "What is your opinion about "clean and unclean foods." I can't tell you that I have come up with a perfect explanation to settle the debate between men who are well studied on both sides of the argument. However, keeping in mind that I have always believed that my spiritual condition will not be affected by what I eat, I have personally decided to "take the path of caution" rather than risk my health.

In the past, whenever anyone talked about dietary habits in reference to the Bible, I thought they were putting us back "under the law." So before we begin any discussion about eating habits, I want to make it perfectly clear that I believe man is not, and never was, made right with God by observing Old Testament food laws. What we eat has absolutely nothing to do with our salvation. Genesis 15:6 says, *"Abram believed the LORD, and he credited it to him as righteousness;"* Hebrews 9:9-10 says, *"The gifts and sacrifices being offered were not able to clear the conscience of the worshiper. They are only a matter of food and drink and various ceremonial washings – external regulations applying until the time of the new order;"* Galatians 2:16 says, *"Know that a man is not justified by observing the law, but by faith in Jesus Christ."*

Dr. Russell, in *What the Bible says about Healthy Living*, supports this truth in his discussion about clean and unclean animals. He says, *"...observing Old Testament ceremonial or dietary laws or secondary Jewish traditions have absolutely no effect on whether we are ceremonially or spiritually clean or unclean* (1996. 12)." The dietary laws have no saving value, but were meant strictly for health.

Jordan Rubin, in *The Makers Diet* agrees with Dr. Russell. He emphasizes the practical purpose of what scripture says concerning food: "God gave His moral law and His dietary guidelines to the Jews at the same time. The moral guidelines preserved spiritual purity, social order, family stability, and community prosperity....Just as the moral guidelines preserved the culture of Israel, so the dietary guidelines preserved their physical health. God's dietary guidelines are not some narrow-minded religious exercise...They were given by a loving God to save His people from physical devastation long before scientific principle of hygiene, viral transmission, bacterial infection, or molecular cell physiology were understood (2004. 35)." What a loving God – full of grace for the weaknesses of man!

In my studies I had to ask myself, "Why is it that I have no problem accepting God's moral guidelines as valid for my moral well-being, but I struggle with the physical benefits of the dietary guidelines." That's where the research in Dr. Russell's book brought scientific clarification. A study was done at Johns Hopkins University by a Dr. Macht who classified animals according to their toxicity to the human body.

All of the animals that God made for food (*clean*) fell into the non-toxic category, while the animals which God did not make for food (*unclean*) fell into the toxic category. Dr Macht's research indicates that what God created for food is healthy, while what He did not create for food is toxic to our bodies. That's why, in our culture, I prefer to use the words toxic or non-toxic instead of clean or unclean. Using these words better defines our purpose which is to achieve healthy dietary guidelines. The chart on the following page lists these foods according to their scientific category.

TOXIC FOODS: What God Did Not Create for Food - Called *Unclean* in Scripture			
(All of these foods have been found to be toxic to man)			
Camel	Leviticus 11:4-7	Cover Fat	Leviticus 3:17
Coney	Leviticus 11:4-7	Blood	Leviticus 3:17
Rabbit	Leviticus 11:4-7	Other Scavenger Animals	Leviticus 11:29,30
Pig	Leviticus 11:4-7	Fish with no fins or scales	Leviticus 11:9,10

These lists are by no means exhaustive, either in a Biblical sense or a scientific sense. I have merely chosen a few to show that what God called *clean* is truly clean and what God called *unclean* is truly unclean.

NON-TOXIC FOODS: What God Clearly Created for Food			
(None of the meats below was listed in Dr. Macht's study as being toxic to our bodies. Quite the contrary, every animal on this list whose blood was tested, was classified as non-toxic.)			
Almonds	Genesis 43:11	Grapes	Deuteronomy 23:24
Barley	Judges 7:13	Grasshoppers, Locusts	Leviticus 11:22
Beans	Ezekiel 4:9	Herbs	Exodus 12:8
Beef	1 Kings 4:22,23	Honey	Isaiah 7:15
Bread	1 Samuel 17:17	Lentils	Genesis 25:34
Broth	Judges 6:19	Meal	Matthew 13:33
Cheese	Job 10:10	Oil	Proverbs 21:17
Vegetables	Numbers 11:5, Proverbs 15:17	Olives	Deuteronomy 28:40
Curds of Cow's Milk	Deuteronomy 32:14	Pomegranates	Numbers 13:23
Figs	Numbers 13:23	Quail	Numbers 11:32
Fish with Fins and Scales	Leviticus 11:9 Matthew 7:10	Raisins	2 Samuel 16:1
Certain Birds	Deuteronomy 14:11	Salt	Job 6:6
Fruit	2 Samuel 16:2	Sheep	Deuteronomy 14:4
Wild Game	Genesis 25:28	Spices	Genesis 43:11
Goat's Milk	Proverbs 27:27	Vinegar	Numbers 6:3
Grain	Ruth 2:14	Wild Honey	Psalm 19:10
Veal	Genesis 18:7,8	Wheat	Psalm 81:16

Note: Some foods mentioned in the Bible have a different meaning than what we apply to them today. For instance, *corn* in the Bible actually refers to grains or seeds. Our type of corn is actually very hard to digest and should be eaten infrequently. *Meat* often refers to ceremonial foods, solid foods, as opposed to milk, or even a portion of food.

In chapter two we discussed 2 principles given by Dr. Russell to guide us in what we should and should not eat. Those 2 principles were:

1. Eat foods as they were created
2. Don't make any food your god.

I mentioned that Dr. Russell has 3rd principle as well. The 3rd principle is:

Eat only what God gave us for food. Following is the reasoning behind this principle.

Eating something other than what God created for food may lead to disease.

Unclean meats which are toxic to the body include black bear, dog, donkey, horse, rabbit, rat, swine, bat, hawk, owl, ostrich, stork, vulture, and fish without scales and fins. The last one really bothered me – I love shrimp and crab legs! Then I learned that these animals are scavengers meant to clean up garbage (including dung and dead animals) from the earth. Their digestive systems aren't designed to get rid of the garbage. Below are just two animals God called *unclean.* I chose these particular two because they're the ones most commonly eaten by us today. I would never think of eating bats or vultures, but I've eaten pork all my life simply because it's part of my culture (I'm originally from Iowa).

Examples of foods listed as toxic by Dr. Russell:

Shellfish filter volumes of water leaving them laden with toxins, harmful bacteria, parasites, viruses, and mercury. Parasites act just like ticks inside our body. All who have had a bacteria or a virus know that they can make you ill. Mercury can cause generally poor health, headaches, fatigue, loss of appetite, decreased sex drive, or poor memory. It may also alter the cell's ability to exchange materials, hinder enzymes, interfere with nerve impulses, cause tremors, depression, and inability to concentrate. The most common thing to which mercury contributes is foggy brain. On the opposite hand, tuna (a clean fish), contains alkylglycerols which pull out toxic mercury and remove it.

Pork contains more toxins than any other meat. They eat anything they can find, including dead animals and their own dung. Dead animals contain parasites, bacteria, viruses and toxins. Since the digestive system of a pig is not designed to excrete these, whatever the pig eats, ends up in anyone who eats the pig. This can lead to blood diseases, stomach disorders, cancer, liver disease, and other illnesses. Note: The digestive system of cows (a *clean* animal) actually crowds out harmful bacteria and parasites.

Cover Fat was not given to us by God for food (Leviticus 4-9). Cover fat was to be burned. As part of God's perfect design, cover fat holds toxins (toxins actually seek out cover fat) and then melts them away. It's interesting that God also designed our cover fat to melt away with proper eating and exercise.

WHAT I CHOSE TO DO: Eat only what God's Word says He created for food. Chelation therapy can be used to remove excess heavy metals from your system. Oral chelation agents can be purchased at your health food store. They include agents which may help with Parkinson's, Alzheimer's, arthritis, and Multiple Sclerosis.

As for Biblical interpretation, please keep in mind that the words clean and *unclean* are used several different ways in scripture. They can be used in a ceremonial sense to refer to whether or not a sacrificial offering was acceptable to God. This of course was taken very seriously by religious leaders of that day. However, they can also be used figuratively, as physical illustration of a spiritual truth.

For instance, the first scripture concerning clean and unclean animals, usually called into question, is found in Acts 10. In this scripture, God seemed to be telling Peter in a vision that He could eat food which had been called *unclean* in Leviticus. First, we must take the scripture in context. In this vision, God's purpose was to tell Peter he could now to go the Gentiles. Up to this time, Gentiles had been called *unclean*, just like food. God had told the Israelites not to become united with the Gentiles so they would not adopt their wicked ways. The question is this: since God was telling Peter he could now go to the Gentiles, does that mean God was also telling Peter he could eat the forbidden foods?

In verse 28, Peter says that God gave him the interpretation of the vision. He says, *"But God has shown me that I should not call any **man** impure or unclean."* Notice that he says man, not animal. The emphasis is on reaching the Gentiles. And the truth is, after the vision, it does not say Peter went and ate the animals in obedience to God. On the contrary, he went to the home of Cornelius to share the gospel. Peter had never eaten the food before the vision, and we have no indication that he did so after the vision.

Beyond this, I would suggest that you read the books written by Dr. Russell and Dr. Rubin, and decide for yourself. Whatever you decide, please **be careful not to judge** other people for what they chose to eat (Romans 14:1-4), and **eat whatever is placed in front of you so as not to insult a host** (Luke 10:8). And above all else, as you follow these guidelines, **do it for the glory of God**, making it your personal goal to achieve better health. You'll be glad you did!

APPENDIX B

SHOPPING LIST FOR THE ONE WEEK MENU AND FOR STOCKING YOUR PANTRY	
I tried to include recipes that do not have unusual items in them. Check to see what you already have on hand. Check off what you already have, and then redo this list according to how your store is arranged.	
Bread	Stone ground whole wheat, Ezekiel bread, whole wheat buns. Trisciuts, Kashi TLC and (New) Breton crackers have no trans fats. La Tortilla wraps have no trans fats.
Condiments	Dijon mustard, Smuckers peanut butter, omega 3 mayo from health food store
Cereal	Old Fashioned Oatmeal, Go Lean, All Bran, Fiber One, Shredded Wheat, Grape Nuts, Granola
Cheese	Feta, goat, grated parmesan
Eggs	2 dozen omega 3 (free range)
Fish	2 fillets (salmon, halibut, or walleye) canned tuna and salmon
Fruit	Fresh: peaches (if planning to top pancakes with them), apples, grapes, mandarin oranges, bananas, melon, strawberries Frozen: mixed berries, blueberries and raspberries, orange juice concentrate, avocado
Herbs and Spices	Italian seasoning, McCormick All Purpose Seasoning (Salt Free), lemon pepper, chives, bay leaves, dried dill and cilantro, sesame seeds, minced onion, cayenne, cinnamon. Any individual seasonings you want to try.
Meat	Buy free range meats. For the first week's menu, you will need 1 LB ground turkey, 6 pieces of chicken on the bone, 2 turkey breasts, 2 lean steaks (preferably free range)
Milk and Dairy	Preferably organic. Natural yogurt (health food store, or Danon natural), cottage cheese, butter (no margarine)
Nuts	Raw almonds and walnuts
Oils	Extra virgin olive oil (expeller/cold pressed), coconut oil
Potatoes	New potatoes
Pasta/ Noodles/Rice	Whole grain or semolina noodles, Near East wild rice and rice pilaf, basmatti rice
Soups and Broth's	If you buy it processed, choose low sodium natural broth which is available at health food stores. I use Swanson's organic boxed broth in a pinch (soup aisle)
Sweets	Honey, raw sugar (at your health food store), Xylo Sweet
Vegetables	Frozen: broccoli, 2 mixed vegetables for soup, sweet pepper medley for soup, sugar snap peas, carrots. Fresh: romaine lettuce, carrots, green beans, red and yellow sweet peppers for salad, sweet pepper for green beans, green beans, cherry tomatoes, mushrooms, 2 bunches of green onions, celery, cabbage, vidallia onion, zucchini, sugar snap peas, garlic cloves, 4 Roma tomatoes, 2 lemons, and cucumbers
Vinegar	Red wine vinegar, apple cider vinegar, soy sauce (low sodium)
Canned foods allowed	Tomatoes, tomato juice, beef and chicken broth (I use Swanson's organic in a box).
Not every town has a health food store, so you may need to make some substitutions.	

APPENDIX C

☐ Fruit ☐ Fruit ☐ Fruit ☐ Fruit	☐ Vegetable ☐ Vegetable ☐ Vegetable ☐ Vegetable ☐ Vegetable	☐ Grains ☐ Grains ☐ Grains	☐ Meat ☐ Meat ☐ Meat	☐ Dairy ☐ Dairy ☐ Dairy	☐ Sat Fat ☐ Omega 3 ☐ Omega 6 ☐ Mono-unsaturated	☐ Herbs ☐ Seeds ☐ Spices ☐ Nuts
☐ Fruit ☐ Fruit ☐ Fruit ☐ Fruit	☐ Vegetable ☐ Vegetable ☐ Vegetable ☐ Vegetable ☐ Vegetable	☐ Grains ☐ Grains ☐ Grains	☐ Meat ☐ Meat ☐ Meat	☐ Dairy ☐ Dairy ☐ Dairy	☐ Sat Fat ☐ Omega 3 ☐ Omega 6 ☐ Mono-unsaturated	☐ Herbs ☐ Seeds ☐ Spices ☐ Nuts
☐ Fruit ☐ Fruit ☐ Fruit ☐ Fruit	☐ Vegetable ☐ Vegetable ☐ Vegetable ☐ Vegetable ☐ Vegetable	☐ Grains ☐ Grains ☐ Grains	☐ Meat ☐ Meat ☐ Meat	☐ Dairy ☐ Dairy ☐ Dairy	☐ Sat Fat ☐ Omega 3 ☐ Omega 6 ☐ Mono-unsaturated	☐ Herbs ☐ Seeds ☐ Spices ☐ Nuts
☐ Fruit ☐ Fruit ☐ Fruit ☐ Fruit	☐ Vegetable ☐ Vegetable ☐ Vegetable ☐ Vegetable ☐ Vegetable	☐ Grains ☐ Grains ☐ Grains	☐ Meat ☐ Meat ☐ Meat	☐ Dairy ☐ Dairy ☐ Dairy	☐ Sat Fat ☐ Omega 3 ☐ Omega 6 ☐ Mono-unsaturated	☐ Herbs ☐ Seeds ☐ Spices ☐ Nuts
☐ Fruit ☐ Fruit ☐ Fruit ☐ Fruit	☐ Vegetable ☐ Vegetable ☐ Vegetable ☐ Vegetable ☐ Vegetable	☐ Grains ☐ Grains ☐ Grains	☐ Meat ☐ Meat ☐ Meat	☐ Dairy ☐ Dairy ☐ Dairy	☐ Sat Fat ☐ Omega 3 ☐ Omega 6 ☐ Mono-unsaturated	☐ Herbs ☐ Seeds ☐ Spices ☐ Nuts
☐ Fruit ☐ Fruit ☐ Fruit ☐ Fruit	☐ Vegetable ☐ Vegetable ☐ Vegetable ☐ Vegetable ☐ Vegetable	☐ Grains ☐ Grains ☐ Grains	☐ Meat ☐ Meat ☐ Meat	☐ Dairy ☐ Dairy ☐ Dairy	☐ Sat Fat ☐ Omega 3 ☐ Omega 6 ☐ Mono-unsaturated	☐ Herbs ☐ Seeds ☐ Spices ☐ Nuts
☐ Fruit ☐ Fruit ☐ Fruit ☐ Fruit	☐ Vegetable ☐ Vegetable ☐ Vegetable ☐ Vegetable ☐ Vegetable	☐ Grains ☐ Grains ☐ Grains	☐ Meat ☐ Meat ☐ Meat	☐ Dairy ☐ Dairy ☐ Dairy	☐ Sat Fat ☐ Omega 3 ☐ Omega 6 ☐ Mono-unsaturated	☐ Herbs ☐ Seeds ☐ Spices ☐ Nuts
☐ Fruit ☐ Fruit ☐ Fruit ☐ Fruit	☐ Vegetable ☐ Vegetable ☐ Vegetable ☐ Vegetable ☐ Vegetable	☐ Grains ☐ Grains ☐ Grains	☐ Meat ☐ Meat ☐ Meat	☐ Dairy ☐ Dairy ☐ Dairy	☐ Sat Fat ☐ Omega 3 ☐ Omega 6 ☐ Mono-unsaturated	☐ Herbs ☐ Seeds ☐ Spices ☐ Nuts

Resource List

Rex Russell, M.D., What the Bible Says About Healthy Living (Ventura, CA: Regal Books, 1996)

Jordan S. Rubin, N.M.D., The Maker's Diet (Lake Mary, Fl: Siloam, 2004)

Jordan S. Rubin, N.M.D., Joseph Brasco, M.D., Restoring Your Digestive Health (New York, NY: Kensington Publishing, 2003)

Don Colbert, M.D., What You Don't Know May Be Killing You (Lake Mary, FL: Siloam, 2004)

Don Colbert, M.D., Toxic Relief (Lake Mary, Fl: Siloam, 2003)

Don Colbert, M.D., The What Would Jesus Eat Cook Book (Nashville, TN: Thomas Nelson, Inc, 2002)

Phyllis A. Balch, CNC & James F. Balch, M.D., Prescription for Nutritional Healing (New York, NY: Penguin Putnam, Inc., 2000)

Ted Boer, M.D., Maximum Energy (Lake Mary, Fl: Siloam, 1999)

Christopher Dobbs, Elson Haas, Vitamins for Dummies (Indianapolis, IN: Wiley, John and Sons, Inc., 1999)

Carol Ann Rintzer, Nutrition for Dummies (Indianapolis, IN: Wiley, John and Sons, Inc., 2003)

Barrie Fox, Nadine Taylor, Arthritis for Dummies (Indianapolis, IN: Wiley, John and Sons, 2000)

Reginald Cherry, M.D., The Bible Cure (San Francisco, CA: Harper, 1999)

Ann Louise Gittleman MS, CNS, The Fat Flush (New York, NY: McGraw-Hill, 2001)

Arthur Agatston M.D., The South Beach Diet (New York, N.Y.: Random House, 2003)

The Reader's Digest Association, The Healing Power of Food (Canary Wharf, London: Readers Digest, 1999)

Ted Broer, Maximum Energy, (Lake Mary, FL: Siloam, 1999)

The Staff of Prevention Magazine, The Complete book of Vitamins (Rodale Press, Inc. 1977)

Mark Bricklin, Rodale's Encyclopedia of Natural Home Remedies (Rodale Press, Inc. 1982)

Gardenoflife.com

DrColbert.com

WestonAPrice.org

Mercola.com

ADDITIONAL RESOURCES FROM TWIFORD MINISTRIES

Where Heaven Meets Earth (Book and Conference)

Loving Your City (Manual and Conference)

Information concerning these resources can be obtained at twifordministries.com or by writing Don at dontwiford@gmail.com or Vicki at vickitwiford@gmail.com.

My Plan for Better Health (summary)

1.   What I need to change about my eating habits

2.   Foods I need to include in my eating habits

3.   Possible choice for cleansing

Additional Notes

Liver Cleanse

Probiotics

Kefir - Stoneyfield

organic
non gmo

Barleans greens -

Traditional Greens Pak - compare to Nixin Red

Dr Steinman - will treat you naturally -

Good Earth - certified -

Don't Stress Diet

FB Eating with Purpose

Tasty Vegetables Plus

Sweet Potatoe Stackers

Coconut oil TB
butter   tsp
drop of almond
drop of stevia

- Grape seed oil -

Beyond Diet

Whole food vitamin
Alive

Unrefined
organic
cold press

Made in the USA
Middletown, DE
16 January 2016